You're So Skinny!

Advice, Personal Life Experiences, and Over 50 Weight Management Tips on Maintaining a Slim Figure

Deninne Jackson

Bloomington, IN  Milton Keynes, UK

authorHOUSE®

AuthorHouse™
1663 Liberty Drive, Suite 200
Bloomington, IN 47403
www.authorhouse.com
Phone: 1-800-839-8640

AuthorHouse™ UK Ltd.
500 Avebury Boulevard
Central Milton Keynes, MK9 2BE
www.authorhouse.co.uk
Phone: 08001974150

First published by AuthorHouse 4/17/2007

ISBN: 978-1-4259-9651-2 (sc)

Library of Congress Control Number: 2007900897

Printed in the United States of America
Bloomington, Indiana

This book is printed on acid-free paper.

Dedication:

I would like to dedicate this book to the following loved ones:

My husband Vince, for being patient with me.

For my son Brandon, who is one of the special loves in my life.

For my best friend in the whole world- Michelle (old faithful), I am so glad to have you in my life.

I would also like to thank my parents, all of my family members and friends for the love that you have shown to me.

God has truly blessed me.

Deninne Jackson

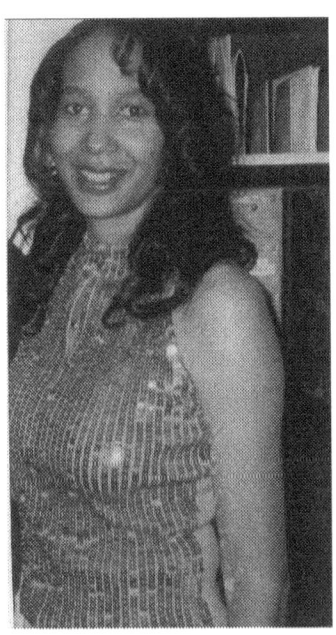

ABOUT THE AUTHOR

Deninne Jackson is a middle-aged, married woman with a ten-year-old son. Mrs. Jackson has been a Human Resource Professional for over thirteen years. She is an entrepreneur, a skillful cook, an avid basketball fan, and very sociable at entertainment events. She participated briefly in a modeling showcase in Hollywood, California, while in college. She also participated in a college-based fashion show. Deninne Jackson has always maintained a tall and slim figure. She has a very youthful appearance and attitude. Her philosophy of life is that if you think and act young, then you will be young. Mrs. Jackson is using her story to inspire others into achieving their personal goals, to bring to light the overweight epidemic that is plaguing the United States, and to provide real and practical solutions towards maintaining an optimum weight level. She discusses the weight management methods that she developed early in life, which led to her long-term success. Her strong spiritual beliefs played an important role in her benefiting physically by applying certain biblical principles to her everyday life. Discipline towards food was self-taught and was also learned by observing friends and relatives with poor eating habits. Many illnesses, such as cancer, diabetes, stroke, smoking addiction, asthma, obesity, gout, drug addiction, and alcoholism, were witnessed firsthand by Mrs. Jackson. This was a deterrent to stay away from unhealthy choices and take care of her body. She has worked as a volunteer in the first annual Asthma Walk-a-Thon in Los Angeles and is a member of the American Lung Association. With long, lean legs, at five feet, nine inches and 129 pounds, Mrs. Jackson's girlish shape rivals that of the supermodels and will make them green with envy.

Disclaimer

This book is designed to provide information on weight management. It is sold with the understanding that the publisher and author are not engaged in rendering legal, medical, or other professional services. If medical, legal, or other expert assistance is required, the services of a competent medical professional should be sought.

It is not the purpose of this guide to reprint all the information that is otherwise available to the general public, but instead to complement, amplify, and/or supplement other fitness and weight management books. You are encouraged to read all the available material, learn as much as possible about nutrition and fitness, and tailor the information to your individual needs.

Contents

CHAPTER 1

My Weight as a Child: It Runs in the Family!

Body Structure and Shape

As a child, I always had a slender shape. It was due, in part, to the fact that I was a picky eater. Being a finicky eater has its advantages.

> **Tip #1** Don't eat what you don't like. This prevents you from over-indulging in food.
>
> **Tip #2:** Only nibble when trying a new food. Don't pile up your plate with new items. Eat only small portions.
>
> **Tip #3:** Eat slowly. Research has shown that it takes approximately eighteen to twenty minutes for food to digest, so by eating slower, you will not eat as much, as opposed to eating faster, which will allow you to consume more food.

Being thin ran in my family. My mother used to tell me stories of how my grandmother would prepare small portions of food on a small plate. In addition, my grandfather lived to be eighty-nine years old and was in relatively good health. He was a thin man, and he also stayed very active during his retirement years. My mother and father were also thin as children and adolescents and into early adulthood. My father used to say that when he first married my mother, she used to eat like a bird.

With that in mind, there is some truth in the saying that you are what you eat, and eating small portions will help to maintain your weight.

All my brothers and sisters were thin growing up as children. We were very active, which included walking to and from school every day. We never skipped breakfast, lunch, or dinner.

> **Tip #4: Eat three small meals per day. Don't skip meals. Don't overeat. Stop eating when you feel full. Do some form of walking every day.**

Some words of advice: Don't stretch your stomach! Don't force yourself or your family to finish everything on their plate. My mom sometimes had a difficult time getting us to eat dinner. She used to have to sit at the table with the belt just to get us to eat. Sometimes I used to put food in my napkin and pretend that I was finished eating. My mom always ensured that we ate complete meals, and she limited our soda intake. We drank a lot of Kool-aid, which is actually lower in calories than soda. When we did drink soda, it was on an occasional basis, and we never went to sleep right away after eating. We used to watch television after dinner, and we were never allowed to eat in our bedrooms.

> **Tip #5: Cut down on the amount of soda you drink. Sodas are higher in calories than Kool-aid, juices, and lower-calorie drink mixes.**

Don't go to bed right away after eating a full meal. Try to do something such as a task or chore or watch TV, but let your food digest before going to sleep. Don't eat food in your bed. This may make you fall off to sleep in your bed immediately after eating. This food will turn into fat and your body will store it.

Family gatherings are also great for trying different types of food! Both my parents and my grandparents loved to participate in family celebrations. Food and dancing were a big part of our family gatherings. There was always plenty of food to feed our large family. Even when we had cousins over for a visit, they would bring their favorite dish or two. We had endless cakes, pies, gumbo, chicken, rice dishes, pasta dishes, vegetables, and all sorts of meat and other food. But you couldn't have a party without dancing. Even then the children and toddlers would dance. After all of the festivities, we always had lots of leftovers. There were times when I didn't like to eat the leftovers. I didn't want to eat the same food that I'd just had the day before. Sometimes I just wanted something light and sweet to snack on. This was where cereal came into play. I like to eat a bowl of cereal as a late-night snack to stop the hunger pangs. Some of my favorite cereals to eat were Cap'n Crunch and Cocoa Puffs, just to name two.

> **Tip #6: After a large meal, try dancing. Put on some music and dance through a song or two. If you get hungry at night, try a light snack or a bowl of cereal to eat.**

My grandmother was a very thin woman; however, she was not happy with her weight. She was born in the early 1900s, and during those times it was more fashionable to have more body fat than to be slender. My grandmother didn't like to cook very much, even though she was not a wealthy woman. This could be one of the reasons why she was so thin. At that time, there were no fast-food establishments for her to order food from for her family. When we were very young, fast-food franchises had just started to open, so my parents took us out to eat on an occasional basis. I guess it was because they had six kids, and it could be very expensive to feed six children.

> **Tip #7: Limit the number of visits you make to eat out at fast-food restaurants. If you do go, then order smaller food combinations, such as a small burger, drink, and fries. They will fill you up just as quickly as a large super-sized combo meal. Don't order combo meals. Your body doesn't need all that food. If necessary, just order a salad, a burger, and a drink and leave out the fries. If you want to order fries and the burger, ask for water as an alternative to soda. This will help you cut down on the number of calories while still being able to eat and enjoy your favorite foods.**

At dinnertime, occasionally, I used to nibble on some candy before dinner to curb my appetite. My favorite candy was banana-flavored

Now-Laters. My mom had to cook large quantities of food for our large family, and it did take a while to prepare and cook. She prepared a variety of meals such as steak, pork chops, roast, chicken, and sausage. We ate a lot of red beans and rice, rice and gravy, and macaroni and cheese. Every Friday, we ate shrimp fried rice and fish as a weekend treat. We generally ate dinner around the same time of the week, including weekends, unless we were out of the house on the weekend. Our lunch consisted mostly of the same thing every day. In high school it was a ham sandwich, some chips, and a piece of fruit such as an orange or an apple. We grew up before juice boxes were popular, so instead of packing sodas, my mother told us that we had to drink water. I used to feel slighted because other kids would drink lots of soda at school; but actually water was better for us in the long run.

Tip #8: Before eating a large meal, try snacking on a few pieces of candy or something sweet. This will give you quick energy from the sugar, and it will cut your appetite, so you will feel less hungry and you will eat less. Try to eat your meals around the same time each day. This will get your body into a set routine, and it will stay on track for meals.

Drink water! Your body needs it and you will flush out your system. My grandfather would participate in many activities. Singing was his favorite pastime. He also enjoyed bowling and going to the movies. I personally enjoy watching comedies. They are definitely a relief from stress, and it is said that laughter burns calories. Both my grandparents, as well as my parents, are from New Orleans, Louisiana. My mom used to tell us that the people who lived down south generally seemed to be more hospitable than people in the western part of United States. She said that she could remember many family gatherings where people would visit each other and bring lots of food to enjoy Sunday suppers. Gumbo and poor boy sandwiches were inexpensive and were also a popular food in Louisiana. Gumbo is mainly a seafood soup served over a bowl of rice, and a poor boy sandwich consists of various meats and cheeses on a long dinner roll. Currently, gumbo and poor boy sandwiches are considered popular specialty dishes throughout the United States.

Tip #9: Try singing or laughing. It is good exercise for the lungs, and it will make you feel better. Watch a funny movie or put on a CD. Laughter is found to be good for the heart. Also, eat soup. Soup is low in calories and very nutritious; however, watch out for the high sodium and preservatives that certain soups contain. Try making your own soup with leftovers. It's an inexpensive alternative to eating out for lunch and dinner.

As a child, I and my brothers and sisters attended a private, Catholic school. At that time, private schools were considered to be better at providing a quality education and discipline than were public schools. However, there will always be misbehaving children in every school system, whether it's private or public. In elementary school, I was a very thin girl. I used to get teased all the time by some of my male classmates. Some of the names they used to call me were "Olive Oil" and "skinny girl." Of course, as a child, being teased would hurt my feelings. No one likes to be teased, so I just ignored them, and eventually I found my own group of friends at school that accepted me regardless of my size. My favorite school activities were in physical education. In high school, I took an interest to roller skating, tennis, and bike riding. During the summer months, every Sunday, my brothers and sisters and I would head to Venice Beach and roller-skate, skateboard or bike-ride on the beach bike route.

Tip #10: Enjoy exercises on the weekends. Bike riding and roller skating are great forms of exercise. Get out of the house more on the weekends. For an hour or two, go to the park or to the beach. There's no cost involved in being outdoors; it will make you feel better and will give you fresh air for your lungs.

My Favorite Foods

Some of my favorite indulgences include waffles, milk and cereal, baby-back ribs, pork chops, and chocolate. In the morning, I enjoy a glass of milk with my breakfast cereal. I feel that milk is important because of the calcium it contains, and it is low in calories. I also like to have a glass of milk with sweets such as a small piece of cake, cookies, and even candy. I love to eat chocolate. My favorite brand of chocolate is Sees Candies, with the nuts and chews selection. It's perfectly alright to eat a few pieces of candy with a glass of milk. Every now and then I will also eat a fried pork chop or have some baby-back ribs. I feel that it's important to treat yourself to some of the foods that you like on an occasional basis. As a child I was never denied any foods, and we were never put on any type of dieting restrictions. You should never deny yourself your favorite foods. However, you should use common sense, and don't overindulge in them. On my waffles, sometimes I will sweeten them with powdered sugar rather than syrup, because powdered sugar is lower in calories than syrup.

> **Tip #11: Try to substitute high fructose corn syrup products with sugar alternatives that are lower in calories. Try powdered sugar, honey or natural jellies and jams, as opposed to syrup.**

Limit the amount of chocolates and drink a glass of milk or water with the sweets or chocolate. Milk is very filling, and it has very little calories. As a child my parents used to take us out on many outings, such as the zoo, theme parks, the Grand Canyon, museums, and plays. We took many road trips over the years. My parents always ensured that either we ate before we went on our trips or my mom would pack food for us eat in the car. We even took a motor home trip to New Orleans one summer vacation. We took a lot of family vacations and trips together. Drive-in movies were my favorite. My mom would pack sandwiches, fry her own chicken, and bring lots of cookies, chips, and Kool-aid, including her own popcorn.

Tip #12: Eat before going out. Try to plan your meals ahead of time before you go on your outings. This saves money and prevents you from overeating at the event or destination. Prepack your own food and try to take it with you. This allows you to select your own food and beverages and watch your calories as well as to eat healthier.

My mom and dad would pack our food and beverages in a cooler, and we would go to the car and eat when we went to theme parks, then re-enter the park, rather than spend a lot of money at the food stands. For some reason as a child, I did not like to eat a lot of mayonnaise. I preferred mustard on my sandwiches. This turned out to be a good thing, because mayonnaise is loaded with fats. When the ice cream truck passed by on our street, I and the children would get all sorts of sweets from it. My favorites were Big Stick and Asteroid popsicles. During the hot summer months, we would sit in the shade and eat our popsicles. My mom tried to make popsicles once, when she bought a popsicle-making set from Tupperware. She would make a really sweet Kool-aid, and then freeze it in those plastic popsicle containers, but it didn't taste quite as good as the popsicles from the ice cream truck.

Tip #13: Try to limit the amount of mayonnaise you consume. It's loaded with fats. Try alternatives as substitutes. A great way to cool off outdoors is to eat nondairy popsicles, instead of drinking soda. You can make your own popsicles with healthier alternatives by using Crystal Light or some other low-calorie juices and drink mixes.

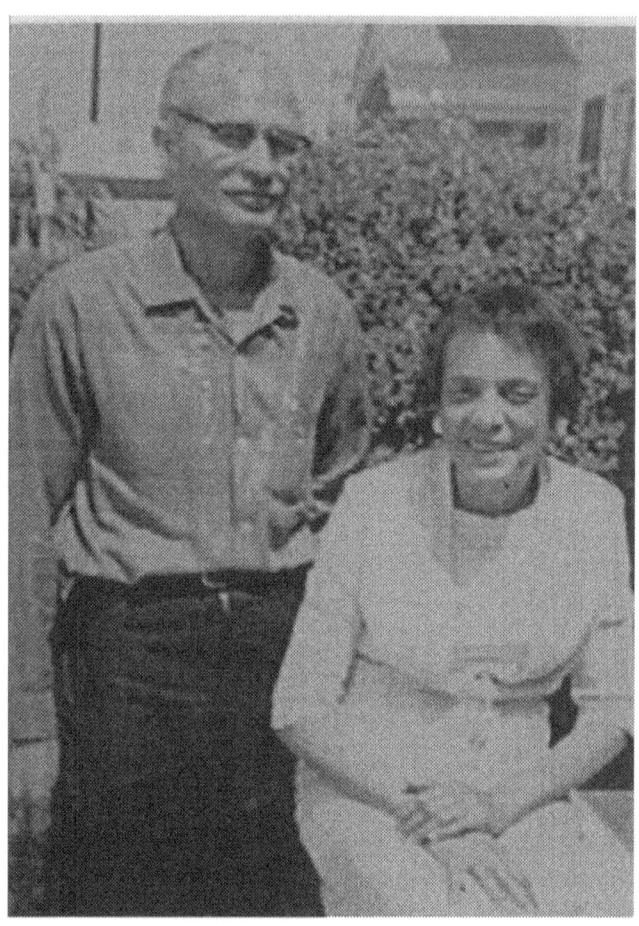

My Grandparents

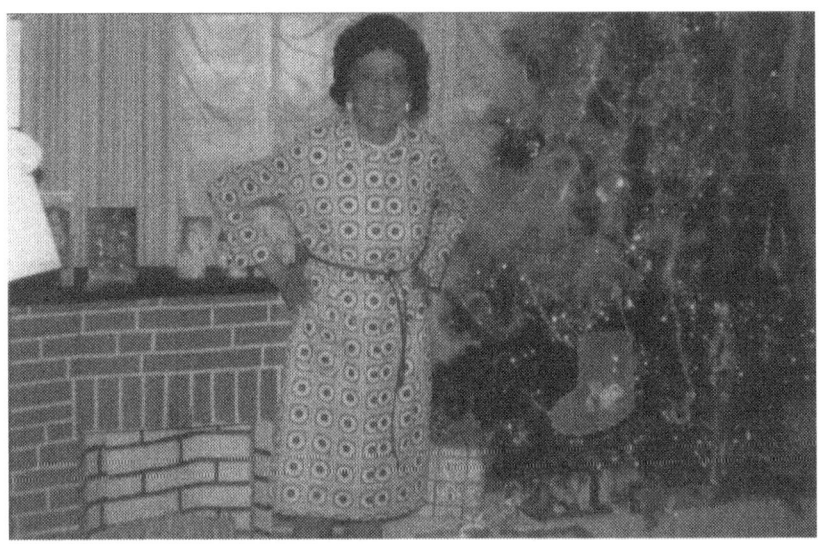

My Grandmother

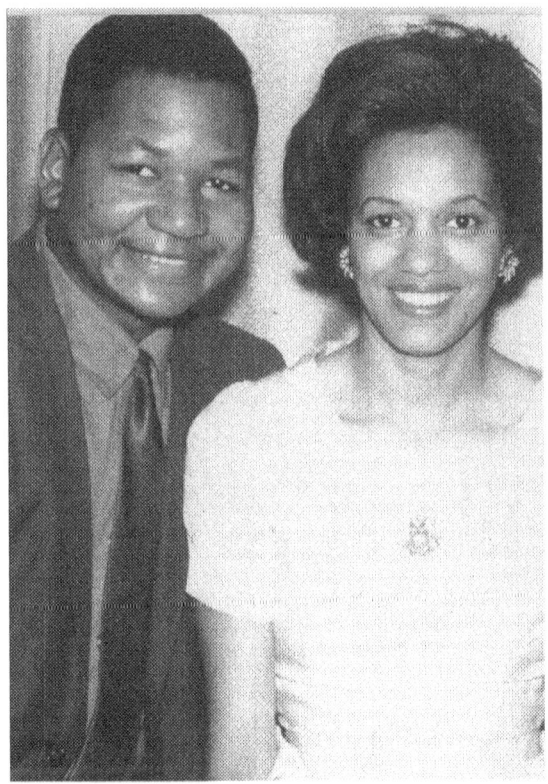

My Mom and Dad

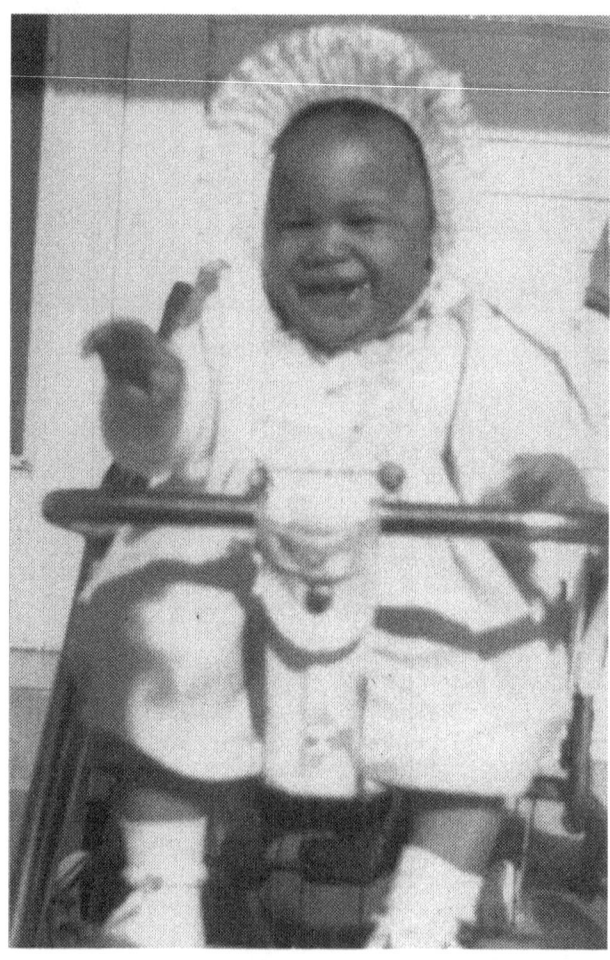

Me as a baby

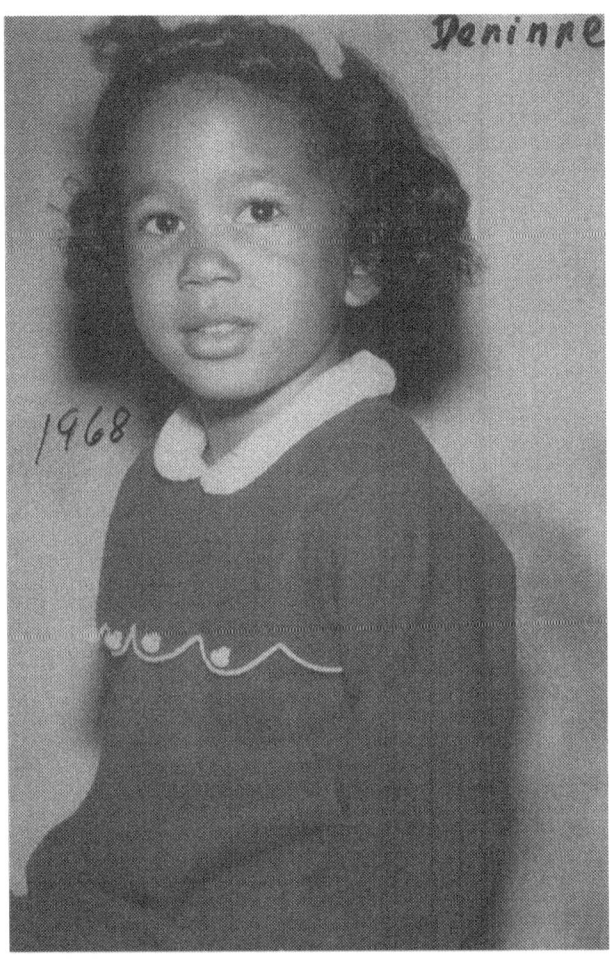

Me as a little girl

CHAPTER 2

Body Image, Body Structure, and Relationships That Impact Eating

I remember in high school, while riding the bus home one day, a male classmate began teasing and taunting me on the bus. An older man interrupted him and said that he shouldn't be behaving in this manner, in front of this young lady (referring to me). My classmate looked at me and said, "Oh she's nobody." The older man told him, she may not be anybody now, but wait until she gets older, she will look great. I always remembered those words as a future compliment, and as I got older, I learned to appreciate my body.

Although I never saw my weight as a problem, I have learned to be confident with my body shape.

Tip #14: No matter what type of body structure you may have, be proud of your shape and don't try to hide it. Confidence makes all of the difference in the world, when people look at you and judge you. Accept your body shape. Wear colors and clothing that accept your body shape. Remember that clothing fads come and go, and not everyone can wear the current fashion trends that come out. Work with clothing that you have and picture how certain styles will look on your body.

I was brought up in a Christian household. Both my parents raised me and my siblings in the Catholic church. I consider myself to be a spiritual person, and I was always taught that your body is your temple. You have to take care of it and not abuse it. What you put into it will determine your overall health and longevity. We were always taught never to smoke cigarettes and never take any illegal drugs.

Tip #15: Don't smoke cigarettes. They are harmful to your body as well as to other people who breathe the smoke. You will pollute your body and you will not reap any benefits from smoking. Don't use any illegal drugs.

Even if you are curious about drugs, never experiment with them. Not only will they cause long-term damage to your body, but they will also destroy your life. My parents felt very strongly against people who smoked. My father said that smoking was a very nasty habit, and he wouldn't allow my grandmother to smoke in our house. My parents also warned us to stay away from people who used drugs. They never associated with people who used drugs. They were very protective parents. We were hardly ever allowed to spend the night over a friend's house if my mother and father did not know her or his parents. My parents were very selective of our friends and who we associated with when we were in high school.

Tip #16: Be careful of the people you associate with, including your friends. If you have friends that may be eating bad or unhealthy foods, are non-supportive or are trying to sabotage your eating plan and living an unhealthy lifestyle, try to limit the amount of time you spend with them. Seek out new friends that you have more in common with towards your weight goals and that are more supportive. It's important to have supportive people in your life. For example, if you are trying to set certain weight goals, and you have friends that are constantly overindulging in their food intake, you may want to pass on some of the invitations, especially when it involves going out to eat.

Tip #17: Limit your sweets at the event or outing and eat before you go out so that you won't overindulge at the event.

Birthday parties are known for having rich cakes and sweet ice cream. If you can't have a small piece of cake, a good option may be to leave the event right at the moment that the cake is being cut. This will also help to fight off any temptations and can avoid packing on some unwanted calories. Change your perception of food: Don't look at it as good food and bad food. Look in the mirror, get a hold of your emotions, and tell yourself that you will not feel guilty if you treat yourself to a favorite food on an occasional basis without overindulging. Tell yourself that you are unique. The most important thing to look at when trying to maintain your ideal weight goal is body image. Body image is basically how you see or picture your own body. It also includes your opinion of how other people observe you. Are you happy with your physical appearance? How do you feel about your body? Are you comfortable in your own body?

I have been working in the human resource field for over thirteen years, with emphasis on employment recruiting. I was very surprised to see over the years the perceptions that hiring managers, including executive staff, have when hiring individuals for a job. People have a lot of biases when it comes to the words "thin" and "fat." There sometimes seemed to have been a negative judgment towards people that were overweight. This perception gave to the managers the impression that the individual may not be quite as productive as a smaller-sized individual. An overweight job applicant was sometimes perceived as not fitting within the company image. Being overweight was sometimes linked with attributes such as laziness, being greedy, unfeminine, sloppy, having personal problems, and being unhappy or even aggressive. On the other hand, being thin was sometimes seen as just the opposite: as being happy, successful, good, strong, feminine, and even confident.

> **Tip #18: Look in the mirror often and tell yourself that you look great!**

Boost your own self-confidence regardless of what other people may say or think. Get a mentor for yourself, or find a motivating factor to help you to succeed in your weight management goals. Take a picture of someone that you admire or desire to look like. Put it on your wall to remind you of your goals on a daily basis. You can also do the same for a particular clothing item that you like.

Use it as a guide to maintain your control and your destiny of where you would like to be. It is also a good idea to fight depression, because this can also hamper your weight goals. Be sure to combat depression and anxiety with positive activities. Since so many people are dissatisfied with their body image, this can be one of the leading causes for depression and anxiety. Sometimes when I am feeling low-spirited, I take my mind off my troubles by reading books or magazines. I also pamper myself with a spa treatment, such as a bath soak or a pedicure.

> **Tip #19: Don't cover up your depression by comforting yourself with food. It's okay to pamper yourself and reward yourself for who you are. You can enjoy your body no matter what size it is.**

Buy a new outfit or do something different, like rent a movie that you would never see at the theatres. A person should never feel guilty about rewarding and treating herself, especially if it is a positive, motivating factor towards meeting her goals. Think positive about your body. I always talk to myself, whether it's having to plan out my day with activities or make phone calls to friends that I have lost contact with. When you talk to yourself, you can build up a positive mental attitude. When you talk to yourself, you can also direct your thoughts and behaviors. If you say to yourself, "I look great in this outfit" or "Stay away from the dessert table," you will have a better chance at success. You have to believe in yourself no matter what your weight goals may be and despite what other people may think or say.

Understanding your body shape and loving your body play important roles in building your self-esteem. A person may think that she is too fat or too skinny, or may want to be taller or shorter or have curly hair, straight hair, a smaller nose, a bigger chest, more muscles, or longer legs. You should never put yourself down. You have to learn how to value yourself and appreciate your own worth. This mindset will greatly play into the way you feel about your body and your determination to do something to change your weight.

> **Tip #20: Take an assessment of your own body. Look at your positive attributes and highlight your best features.**

If you have long legs, choose pants or skirts that maximize the length of your legs. If you have short legs, you can maximize the length of your legs by wearing shorter skirts or higher heels. (This will give the illusion of adding length to your body.) There is a lot of clothing that a person can wear to accentuate her body assets. For example: Biker shorts can be worn by anyone. You don't have to have the perfect body to wear them; you just have to make them fit with the body you have. If you have a large stomach and a large rear end, you can wear a large, oversized T-shirt to cover those body parts and just have your lower legs exposed.

If you are extremely thin, take the large shirt and stuff it into your shorts for the illusion of looking bigger, and wear a form-fitting shirt on top of the large shirt, so that you won't look like the shirt is overtaking your upper body. Relationships can also affect your self-esteem and body image. Over the years I was involved in a few unhealthy relationships. During one previous relationship, I had to deal with anger, various emotions, and jealousy. When I'm feeling down, I can suppress my appetite for longer periods of time, which can cause me to lose weight. This type of unhealthy relationship can cause depression. Unhealthy relationships can affect a person's ability to have a positive body image. It can also lead to overeating at times, as well as undereating.

Everyone has to remember that their self-worth must come from themselves. It should not come from others. Even the behavior of an abuser can sometimes be mistaken for intense feelings of caring or concern. A healthy relationship has trust and respect, and it doesn't mean that you are constantly worried about breaking up in the relationship.

Tip #21: Recognize the fact that you deserve the right to be treated with respect and dignity and should not be physically or emotionally mistreated by another individual.

Trust your intuition. If something does not feel right in the relationship, it probably isn't. If you are suffering from any type of abuse or if you can't love someone without feeling afraid, then you should get out of the relationship quickly. There are many resources, such as counselors, doctors, family members, and friends, that will help you to get out of an unhealthy relationship.

General statistics show that the existing stereotypes of body images that are set for women are far more distorted than the stereotypes of body images that are set for men. Over the years there have been several research studies showing that girls and women generally participate in more appearance-related activities than do their male counterparts; however, the reports also show that men usually gravitate more towards weight training and steroids than do women. The biggest difference between the sexes is that women and girls tend to diet, count calories, and weigh themselves more, are more worried about being overweight, and experience more anxiety and guilt about their looks than do boys and men.

Our body image can be changed by our thoughts and actions. For example, it can change after eating a bowlful of ice cream or after looking at your weight on a scale or hearing some harsh comments about what you're wearing. A woman's body image is fragile and can be affected by negative thoughts such as "I wish I were younger," "I wish I were taller, thinner, or better looking." It's important to have a positive body image. In order to change your negative thoughts into positive thoughts, you need to reinforce your positive behavior in action.

Tip #22: Do not weigh yourself on the scale every day. Put your scale out of sight. Allow room for body changes daily, and for your weight to fluctuate. Some days your skirt or pants will feel tighter. That's OK; use this as an indicator to become more active.

If you are obsessed with your weight and it seems to be hurting your professional as well as your personal life, seek professional counseling. Most employers offer an employees assistance program (EAP), which provides free or low-cost professional face-to-face counseling for employees.

With body image, the true picture that we see may be very true, or it can be distorted. Someone that has gained a lot of weight is surprised to see herself in a window or mirror because the picture She has in her mind is actually the body she had when she was smaller. When an overweight person loses a substantial amount of weight, she can still see herself as being obese.

Tip #23: Look at your body in your mind. Close your eyes and visualize your body and then ask yourself to feel and think about your own body image. For me, I think of myself as a child of God. I am very spiritual, and my body is my temple.

When I think of my body as a special gift, it gives me a positive self-image and body image. My body in my mind has been through a lot of stress, so I know that I have to take good care of it and be kind to it, especially if I want to get the most out of it in my daily routine. I try to eat sensibly, stay active, get plenty of rest, and heal and nourish my body. We can make the aging process much easier if we take a positive attitude and think of our bodies as precious temples.

CHAPTER 3

Eating for Pleasure or Eating to Stop the Hunger?
Food Disorders, Food Cultures, and Food Addictions

Regular eating habits should be an enjoyable and positive experience. Regular eating habits should be flexible and rely on a person's internal signals of thirst, hunger, and fulfillment. Your eating habits develop from your own confidence and trusting yourself to believe that you are eating in a way that's practical for you. This is based on how you feel and your own common sense. Regular eating allows you to eat without guilt, because you are depressed, bored, or happy, or just for pure satisfaction. It also means eating on a consistent basis.

Most of the time, it can also mean having the ability to nibble at a party or eating more now because the food is hot and fresh. Regular eating can be overeating sometimes or feeling full and stuffed. It is also undereating sometimes because you are sick or too busy. Basically regular eating is flexible and guiltless and balances foods by weighing the high calories and fat of some against the lower calories and fat of others. This is all part of a regular eating pattern.

> **Tip #24: Eat your meals from a small plate. If you purchase dessert-sized plates, or even smaller, you are less likely to pile up your plate with too much food.**

I like to use the space rule. Give each food item a little space on your plate. Don't overlap the food and try not to let the food items touch each other. This forces a person to put smaller portions of food on his plate, if he follows this simple rule. Since eating is such a pleasurable experience, it can also have an adverse effect on some people, causing them to become addicted to food.

What is food addiction? Food addiction is when a person can't take control over her craving for food. I'm not just talking about when a person gets the munchies or an occasional snack attack. It's when a person can't function without a chocolate bar, cappuccino latte, soda, or other snack on a daily basis. I absolutely love chocolate, whether it's a candy bar, cup of hot chocolate, ice cream, or cereal. I love the rich flavor that chocolate has, and it also wakes up my senses. I also know that too much of any food, including chocolate, is not good for the body. So, I can go without chocolate. I don't need it to start or end my day. However, a food addict consumes so much of a particular food item that it can lead to certain health risks, such as obesity, high blood pressure, diabetes, and others.

There are various types of food addictions, which lead to specific types of food dependency. One type of food addiction is to sweets or sugars. By eating too many sweets or sugars, you will hinder the body from producing glucose. So if someone is frequently eating sugars or sweets, then her body will constantly rely on the sugar or sweets for energy, as opposed to natural sugars found in carbohydrates. Another type of food addiction is to caffeine. Caffeine is a stimulant and affects the central nervous system. It is found in coffee, tea, chocolate, and even certain sodas. Specialty coffees such as a cappuccino, latte, and espresso also contain caffeine, which is the main reason why some people may need their daily cup(s) of java in the morning, afternoon, and/or evening.

Another type of food addiction is to chocolate. Chocolate contains a chemical called theobromine, which works similar to caffeine. Chocolate is also a stimulant which affects a person's mood. Some women have claimed that chocolate alters their mood so much that it creates a feeling that is better than sex. Chocolate can be found in almost any food, such as cookies, candy, drinks, cereal, etc.

These are just some of the more common food substances that can lead to food addiction. An individual can be addicted to almost any type of food. To find out if you're a food addict, listed are some simple signs that you should be aware of:

- Constant eating
- Insatiable cravings for certain foods
- Weight gain
- Depression or feeling tired
- Still feeling hungry after eating certain foods
- Having withdrawal symptoms
- Having mood swings when hungry

The following are some tips that a person can use to avoid food addiction and food dependency.

Tip #25: **Be aware of how your body reacts to certain foods, especially if you have any unusual cravings and/or withdrawal reactions.**

Tip #26: **See a nutritionist or food counselor if you feel that your eating habits are getting out of control.**

Tip #27: **Don't use food as a comforter. Overeating, a.k.a "pigging out," to ease the pain of loneliness, depression, and low self-esteem can give a false sense of coping and instant gratification, which only masks emotional issues.**

As a teenager, I used to enjoy baking. I took a cooking class in high school, so I began baking cakes and cookies. I used to enjoy licking the spoons and bowls after baking. I had an incredible urge to taste the cake batter and the cookie dough batter. Eventually, as I grew older, I didn't have that much time for baking and thus the urge to eat raw cookie dough went away.

In today's society, eating raw cookie dough has become so popular that it has become a flavor of ice cream that's much in demand. So, you see, eventually any type of food can be addictive. The key factors to remember are to use moderation and be aware of what you eat. Food addiction is a real serious problem. Experts say that over 60 percent of Americans are overweight, which can cause some very serious health problems. The most important thing to remember is that this condition can be treated.

Food and Culture

For millions of people around the world, food plays a vital role and has different meanings (some even being symbolic) in different cultures. More than half of the Southeast Asian population is agriculture based. Twice as much fish is consumed in this region compared with other forms of animal protein. The staple food throughout the region is rice. Rice serves as the basic food for more than half the world's population today. Simple daily meals and elaborate feasts characterize all Southeast Asian culinary cultures.

Cooking is economically efficient, as people use wok cooking, which requires a low amount of fuel and makes deep-frying easy. Also meat and vegetables are typically chopped into small pieces prior to cooking, which means that food cooks very quickly. Most food is cooked by quick blanching or stir frying and steaming. Southeast Asians are concerned with nutrition, economy, and ease of preparation as it relates to their food. With high nutrients, rice is a good source of insoluble fiber, which is also found in whole wheat, brand, and nuts. Insoluble fiber reduces the risk of bowel disorders and fights constipation. Among other nutrients, rice is rich in carbohydrates, the main source of energy, low in fat, and contains some protein and plenty of B vitamins.

Those looking to reduce their fat and cholesterol intakes can turn to rice because it contains only a trace of fat and no cholesterol. Rice is also gluten free, so it is suitable for coelics, and easily digested, and therefore is a wonderful food for the very young and the elderly. Rice is also suitable for vegetarians and vegans, with brown rice in particular complementing vegetarian and vegan dishes. Growing up I can remember that my mother prepared a lot of dishes with rice. One popular dish was red beans and rice.

We also ate many rice and gravy dishes for dinner and egg and rice for breakfast. Every Friday my mother would order shrimp fried rice, which is still one of my favorite dishes today. Rice is a popular dish that is also used in a lot of my Creole family, New Orleans style meals. It is used in gumbo, jumbalaya, dirty rice, and other popular dishes. Although these dishes were part of our New Orleans heritage, they also contained health benefits as well. Rice can be made into a variety of dishes. It can be served with the main dish or made as an appetizer, a drink, or even as a dessert. Rice is an important part of a balanced diet.

The key to maintaining or losing weight is watching the calorie counts in your favorite foods. Portion control involves understanding the serving sizes and the calories associated with them and knowing when and how much to cut back. The following tip can help identify proper portion size.

> **Tip #28:** Three ounces of meat, poultry, or fish is about the size of a woman's palm or a deck of playing cards. One half cup of fruit, vegetables, rice, or pasta is about the size of a small fist. One cup of milk, yogurt, or chopped fresh greens is about the size of a small hand holding a tennis ball. An ounce of cheese is about the size of your thumb tip. By remembering these portion sizes and including rice in your diet, you can prepare a variety of dishes without sacrificing taste in your meals.

There are several differences in European dining norms versus American dining norms. A few of the noted differences are that Europeans hardly ever use ice in their drinks, nor do they usually butter their bread (it tastes good enough on its own). In many countries, every dish is served on a separate plate, so don't expect a little pile of vegetables to come automatically next to your steak.

The salad comes at the end of the meal, before dessert (which makes a lot more sense digestively). You can't take it with you. Europeans don't allow you to take home a doggy bag, and many will be highly confused if you point to your half-eaten plate and ask for the balance of your meal to go—especially if you use the term "doggy bag."

Over the years, there have been many comical exchanges between American diners and European servers, who either are (A) dumbfounded as to why you don't wish to finish your dinner in the restaurant, (B) insulted when they mistake your intentions to be a belief that their fine cooking is only good enough for your dog, or (C) horrified and disgusted as they hasten to assure you that food comes from a cow, not from a dog.

Many Eastern cultures serve several main dishes as part of their dining experience, and consumers are expected to eat everything on their plates, otherwise it is insulting to the host. Wine in France is customary with meals. You should not refuse wine, just sip it slowly.

In France, the wine is carefully picked so that it will complement your food, and sometimes the wine will even change during your meal and dessert. As in Chinese tradition, be careful not to add salt and pepper or any type of spice into your food. It is considered to be insulting to your host. The French believe in smaller portions of food, but with a large number of courses. If you are in a French restaurant, it is expected that you eat and finish everything on your plate.

This is to refrain from asking for seconds. If you are in a French restaurant, you can ask for more water with your food, but you can not ask for more wine. If you want more wine, you are supposed to wait for your host to serve you; and if you are hosting, you must make sure that the glasses of your guests are filled at all times. The French take much pride in the food that they make and process. Eating well is a priority throughout the country. French food uses some of the world's finest seafood, which is the influence of the Alsace. If you move farther down the countryside, typical fare includes fine cheese, meats, bread, vegetables, and herb dishes.

CHAPTER 4

Stay Active! Stay Busy!
Walking, Race Walking, Swimming, and Depression All Impact Food
and Beverage Consumption

Walking is the most important form of exercise. By walking, an individual can have a happier and healthier lifestyle. It is very inexpensive, safe, and easy. Walking can be very relaxing and it can also increase your energy at the same time. Walking does not require a lot of athletic ability, it is not necessary to join a health club, and you do not need to purchase any special equipment other than comfortable and supportive shoes.

Growing up as a child, both myself and my brothers and sisters had to walk to and from school every day. The elementary school was approximately three blocks away from our home. The walking was necessary because my mother had to work, but it was also good for us. It gave us great exercise. There are many benefits and rewards that a person receives from walking. You can gain a more fit and trim body that will allow you to add more years to your life and give you better overall general health. There's a new trend going on all over the nation called "fundamental walking," also known as health walking. This can be done at any time, anywhere, all year round—walking to the park, mall, movies, store, around your neighborhood, with a friend, your dog, alone, and at your own pace.

Walking is easy physical fitness that can be done at your own leisure. Most everyone benefits from walking, regardless of their age. Approximately 67 million people are walking on a regular basis, because they know that it is good exercise, and they are making it a part of their daily routine. According to the President's Council on Physical Fitness and Sports, the numbers are increasing every year.

> **Tip #29: For individuals who have had long periods of inactivity, walking is a great way to start an exercise program. Start slowly, and then build up your speed so you can maintain a steady pace.**

Most podiatric and family physicians recommend walking to help ease or stop many physical ailments. The benefits of walking include strengthening your heart and lungs and improving circulation. It can help to prevent heart attacks and strokes. Walking can reduce obesity and high blood pressure, boost your metabolic rate, and help with your cholesterol. It can improve muscle tone in your legs and abdomen, as well as reduce stress and tension. Walking can also reduce arthritis pain and stop bone tissue decay.

> **Tip #30: When walking, be sure to move at a steady pace, brisk enough to make your heart beat faster. Make sure that you breathe deeply as you walk. Before you begin walking, do some slow and easy warm-up exercises. This will get your muscles to relax and make them more flexible. Good warm-up exercises include touching your toes, knee-bends, and body twists at the waist, in a slow hula-hoop motion. The best way to begin your walking program is to start walking for twenty minutes without interruption at least three times a week. Walk at a pace that is comfortable to you, and slow down if you find yourself breathing heavily. Don't overwork yourself. If you find that twenty minutes is too much, then decrease your walking time to ten or fifteen minutes. You can slowly increase your time and your pace as your body adapts to the walking.**

Tip #31: Keep an activity log, in which you write down the dates, times, and estimated distances of your walks, plus other notes, such as routes, milestones, and incidental experiences. Reading this activity log daily can let you see your progress, and it can also be used as a motivating factor for walking. If you're occasionally uninspired or feel like you're stuck in a rut, change your routine.

My parents used to take us to the beach on Sundays and we would walk all over the sand for miles. We used to look for seashells, and sometimes we would walk for over half an hour on the beach, collecting them. This was great exercise. Walking in sand builds muscles because you have to lift your legs with greater strength because of the resistance of the sand as it pulls downward.

Tip #32: Change your routine. If you get bored with your walking program, try a new class, such as aerobics, kickboxing, salsa lessons, etc. Many different classes are offered during the week at local city recreation centers and colleges. Some even offer weekend classes. Walking and exercising with someone can make the difference between quitting and sticking with a fitness plan. It is best to find someone who is fitter than you are. Research has shown that when someone chooses an exercise or walking buddy that is more physically in shape than she; she will do better and stick to her walking and exercise program. This sort of mentor or buddy can provide you with much needed exercise advice. You will perform much better than when you exercise or walk alone. This buddy or mentor can also help you develop an exercise plan that makes sense and can give you the added push you need.

Should you see a doctor? If you do not have any serious health problems, then you can begin walking with confidence. Walking is not hard work and generally does not cause any serious health risks. One thing to keep in mind is to make sure that you use common sense. Don't push your body beyond its limitations. Be careful not to walk outdoors during extreme weather conditions until you have a good walking program in place. Before beginning any type of walking program, you should consult your family or podiatric doctor. Getting a physical is strongly recommended, especially if someone is over sixty, has a disability or disease, or is taking any kind of medication. It is also a good idea for those individuals who are between the ages of thirty-five and sixty, who are considerably overweight, excessive smokers, or easily fatigued, or who have been physically inactive, to get a physical.

> **Tip #33:** Choose a good-quality, lightweight walking shoe that has breathable upper material, made from leather or nylon mesh. Make certain that the heel is close to the ground, for better walking stability. Fit is very important, so make sure that you get the proper width and good arch support.

Race walking is a great form of exercise. It is a specialized technique that is used by walkers as a form of fitness, as well as for competition. It gets better results than health walking because it is faster and it also increases the heart rate.

As a child, I can recall getting several presents of sporting equipment for Christmas. My parents gave me and my siblings various outdoor gifts, which included bicycles, jump ropes, skates, hula-hoops, footballs, basketballs, tennis racquets, softballs, etc. My mother constantly encouraged us to get out of the house and play, especially on the weekends. With six children, my mother had to make sure that we all stayed active and healthy. This also gave her some free time and quiet time, because she really needed it. I enjoyed many activities, and what was very beneficial to me growing up was having a recreational park right at the corner of my street. The park was a great place to swing or play on the playground. With a park nearby, my family had many birthday parties and picnics there. We were always encouraged to bring our bikes and skates.

Whether you have children or not, a good way to stay active is by bringing a friend or family member to a park, or babysitting for someone that you know and bringing their children to the park.

Swimming is also a great form of exercise and it's very important that everyone, regardless of age, learn how to swim. Although swimming is a seasonal activity, you can find many indoor, heated, year-round pools that allow individuals to take swimming lessons or do some recreational swimming. There are many health benefits of swimming. Swimming uses almost all the major muscle groups and places a vigorous demand on your heart and lungs. Swimming develops muscle strength and endurance and improves posture and flexibility. Swimming is especially useful for people who are overweight or pregnant or have leg or lower back problems. Swimming is also a great sport for people of all ages and all proficiency levels. Swimming provides most of the aerobic benefits that running does, and with many of the benefits of resistance training thrown in.

Swimming, however, does not put the strain on connective tissues that running, aerobics, and some weight training regimens do. Swimming for fitness is rapidly gaining in popularity because it is ideal for almost anyone from competitive types to the physically challenged. Whether you swim laps or do aerobics in the shallow end, swimming is an ideal exercise. Aquatic exercise and therapy are used to treat and prevent physical ailments.

In addition to its therapeutic role, there are several aquatic activities that are very popular for recreational purposes. An individual's ability to swim and feel comfortable in the water creates opportunity to get involved in other water sports, such as kayaking, canoeing, sailing, and water skiing. The buoyancy factor makes swimming the most injury-free sport there is. Water exercise benefits seniors, pregnant women, arthritis sufferers, and anyone with an injury. One of the biggest advantages is flexibility. In water, body weight is one-tenth of what it would be on land. For example, if you weigh 150 pounds on land, then you would weigh fifteen pounds standing in chin-deep water; hence, range of motion in water is much easier. Also, fitness exercise in water can be done more often because of the low incidence of high-impact injuries and is more effective. Before you jump up and go to the pool to swim, there are many things that you should be aware of. Swimming must be done very carefully. Jumping in a pool and swimming laps does not mean that you won't put your health at risk.

> Tip #34: Get a swimming routine to be an important part of
> your exercise process. You should start off with easy breathing
> exercises and learn basic strokes. This will enable you to begin lap
> swimming.

Swimming on a regular basis, even of moderate intensity, can
help reduce high blood pressure in some people. Movement in water
has twelve times greater resistance than movement in air. For pregnant
women, water exercise strengthens and tones the muscles used during
childbirth. For the elderly, water fitness is safe, fills the need for exercise,
increases a body's range of motion, and is a low-impact exercise. For those
with weight problems, water helps the body naturally rid itself of excess
water and salt. As physical therapy, it gradually and gently rehabilitates
and relaxes muscles and joints that have stiffened or atrophied. It is very
important to establish what level of swimmer you are before starting
your swimming exercises.

> Tip #35: At the beginning level, you should focus on the strokes
> and how to breathe while swimming. This is very important,
> as it can prevent you from drowning in the future. Leisurely
> laps are especially good for those who need to exercise slowly.
> By augmenting laps with floats and other swimming aids, even
> beginning swimmers can start making progress at little risk.

> Tip #36: When swimming laps, in either shallow or deep water,
> make certain that you are not the only one in the swimming pool
> or near the pool alone.

Cramps, muscle strains, and other injuries can happen to anyone,
even the professional swimmer. Even though it may be unlikely, it is not
a risk you should take. Growing up, my mother and father would take
me and my brothers and sisters to swimming lessons every summer at
the local park. We started at the park in the mornings, even when it was
cold and the sun wasn't out. This particular park didn't have a chlorinated
pool; it was more of a man-made lake, with a section of it roped off for the

ducks to swim in. I remember that the water was kind of a murky green color and the bottom surface of the lake was sort of slippery.

After a while, we began to take lessons at the local community college pools and public city pools. My point is that you do not have to spend a lot of money to enjoy the great exercise benefits of swimming. My family made swimming a complete family activity. When I was a child, I can remember my entire family driving out to my aunt's house, two hours away, near San Bernardino, and we would go to the local swimming pool. All of my cousins enjoyed swimming. It was a great way to get the entire family together and participate in an activity while having fun at the same time.

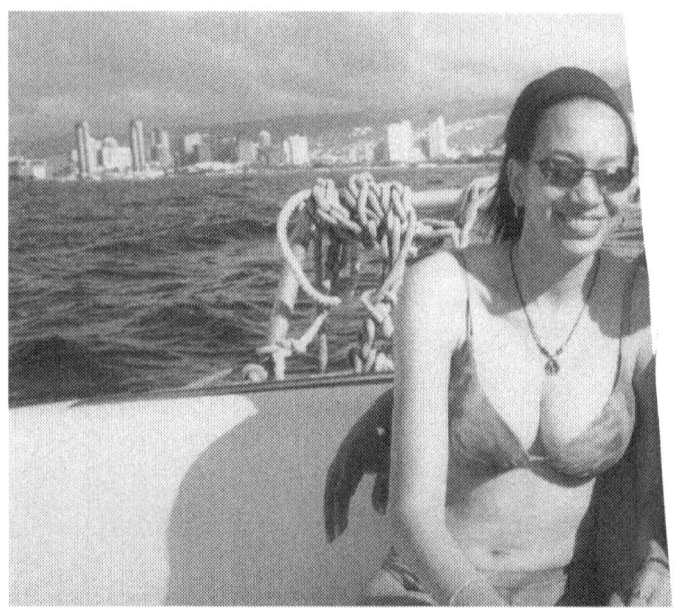

On vacation in Hawaii

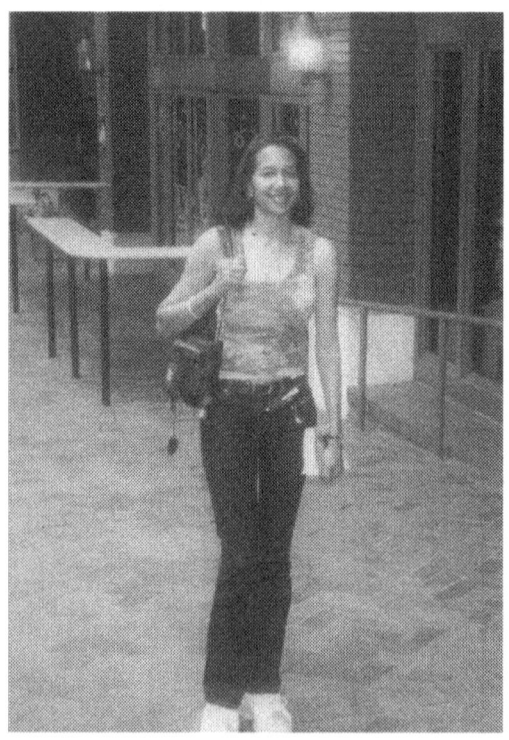

Shopping in Atlanta, GA.

CHAPTER 5

Media Perceptions of Being Beautiful That Can Affect Your Eating Habits

There are numerous studies that discuss the implications of a global society that narrowly defines beauty by the images seen in entertainment, advertising, and fashion runways and the startling impact this has on women. One of the results found was that only 2 percent of thousands of women from ten countries around the world consider themselves beautiful. Does this mean that we live in a world where women are not beautiful, or does it mean that women around the world are calling for a broader definition of beauty? This study also uncovers that beauty is never going away and has enormous power. Beauty should not be reduced to a political or cultural problem, but should be understood as basic human pleasure. The study uncovers the startling information about how women physically perceive and define their look. Supporting the current and narrow definition of beauty, the respondents are hesitant to claim ownership of the word "beauty." More than 40 percent strongly agreeing that they do not feel comfortable describing themselves as beautiful. Furthermore, only 5 percent feel comfortable describing themselves as pretty and a mere 9 percent feel comfortable describing themselves as attractive. Additionally, just 13 percent of women say they are very satisfied with their beauty; 12 percent say they are very satisfied with their physical attractiveness; 17 percent are very satisfied with their facial attractiveness; and only 13 percent are very satisfied with their body weight and shape.

In fact, in a society captivated by diet makeover programs, a third of women around the world are very or somewhat dissatisfied with their body weight. The women of Japan have the highest levels of dissatisfaction, at 59 percent, followed by Brazil (37 percent), United Kingdom and the United States (each at 36 percent), Argentina (27 percent), and the Netherlands (25 percent).

Having assessed how women think about as well as evaluate their own beauty and appearance, the study asks women about social issues emerging from mass media and pop culture. From Brazil to the Netherlands to Argentina—across cultures, ages, ethnicities, and races—women make it clear that they believe that there is a one-dimensional and narrow physical definition of beauty. The findings show that the ideas of beauty and physical attractiveness are largely synonymous, and although both are highly valued by society, both are rendered almost impossible to attain. Respondents said that they felt pressure to try and be that "perfect" picture of beauty. Sixty-three percent strongly agree that women today are expected to be more attractive than their mother's generation. Sixty-six percent strongly agree that society expects women to enhance their attractiveness.

Forty-five percent of women feel that women who are more beautiful have greater opportunities in life. More than half (59 percent) strongly agree that physically attractive women are more valued by men. The study also explores the degree to which mass media has played a role in portraying and communicating a narrow definition of beauty: More than two-thirds (68 percent) of women strongly agree that the media and advertising set an unrealistic standard of beauty that most women can't ever achieve. Well over half of all women (57 percent) strongly agree that "the attributes of female beauty have become very narrowly defined in today's world." The traditional definition of beauty, based only on physical appearance, is powerfully communicated through the mass media and has been assimilated through popular culture. It is this ideal that many women measure themselves against and aspire to attain. However, women around the world would like to see media change in the way it represents beauty. For example, women feel they are surrounded and bombarded with images that are unrealistic: The majority (76 percent) wishes that female beauty were portrayed in the media as being made up of more than just physical attractiveness. Seventy-five percent went on to say that they wish the media did a better job of portraying women of diverse physical attractiveness, including age, shape, and size.

As a young teenager, I can remember a time when I wanted to start wearing makeup to improve my appearance. I saw a photograph of Diana Ross in a magazine, with lots of makeup on and so I tried to imitate her look. I remember going to the grocery store with my mother, however she didn't seem to notice that I had on some blush makeup. When we got to the checkout counter, my older sister said that I had on too much blush and that I looked like a clown. I got angry and then I decided to ignore her. The cashier, who was an older lady, looked at me with sympathy and said, "She's right, honey, it's too much makeup for you." After that embarrassing moment, I stayed clear of blush and I very seldom use it to this day.

Looking back on this situation made me realize that no matter what someone looks like, they always want to look better.

Tip #37: You can create a slimmer image by maintaining good skin care habits and a great haircut/hairstyle and by applying specific makeup techniques to create and enhance an image of thinness in the face.

There are lots of computer software programs on the market to create a computerized or simulated photograph of a person with different types of hairstyles and wearing various shades of makeup. These are virtual hairstylist, virtual makeover, or virtual haircut programs. They allow a person to experiment with different looks before she actually has the work done in a salon. Even though all hair colors and cuts are beautiful, they may not appear beautiful on you. So, when coloring, highlighting, or cutting your hair, carefully consider which shades or cut will flatter your skin tone and body type. A good hairstylist can replicate any style you throw at him or her, but is it realistic for you? Before selecting a style, take into account your hair texture, length, and health and how much time you want to spend styling it each day. "If you're not realistic before you get a haircut, you'll end up being a slave to your hairstylist."

Healthy-looking skin can also create a slimmer image, in the facial area. The face is a very important part of the body and it usually is the first thing that people see and notice on someone before they look at her body. Like it or not, your skin will be with you for the rest of your life. Your skin serves you and your body in a number of ways. It aids in sensory perception, protects you from injuries, provides a barrier against dehydration, assists in temperature maintenance, removes toxic wastes, aids in the manufacture of vitamin D, and provides structure to the organs and tissues within your body. To put it lightly, your skin is an integral part of your life. It's essential that you care for it and maintain it in a healthy state so that it will continue to function well for you as you age.

It is also important that you protect your skin. The ultraviolet rays of the sun are damaging to your skin and to your health. Sun exposure can lead to premature aging, sagging, wrinkles, skin discoloration, and the development of cancer. And while a suntan will eventually fade at the end of summer, the damage to the skin from sunlight will continue to accumulate over time. Take measures to protect your skin from the sun and its damaging rays.

Tip #38: Sunscreen with an SPF (Sun Protection Factor) of at least 15 helps block the damaging rays of the sun and should be used every day for adequate protection. After sun protection, proper skin cleansing is the next best thing you can do for the care and protection of your skin. Choose a gentle skin cleanser based on your skin type and special skin care needs and wash your skin as necessary to keep it clean, fresh, and functioning properly.

Skin care moisturizers smooth and soften skin and help to lock in its natural moisture. Your skin also needs a good balance of vitamins, minerals, and nutrients in order to function and remain healthy. Adequate exercise helps improve circulation and move waste and nutrients through your system. Eat a healthy diet and get plenty of exercise to keep your skin and the rest of your body in tip-top condition.

Tip #39: Drink at least six to eight glasses of purified water throughout the day to hydrate the skin and circulate essential nutrients. Get a shower filter to filter out the harmful chemicals from your city water supply.

The environment in which women learn about the politics of the body is saturated with media presentations of what a woman's body should be. Women in the media are portrayed in terms of their bodies far more than men. Women are judged by more exacting physical and sexual standards even though these standards are often based on images that are airbrushed, enhanced by computer, or trimmed with scissors. Advertisements are highly gendered. It is also important to ask the question of how the dominant images of beauty in the United States affect or do not affect the experiences of women of color versus white women and their attitudes toward the body.

One finding suggests that black women may not be responding to dominant white ideals of beauty in the same way as are white women. In other words, research based on white participants as indicating those white women's perceptions of themselves as "too fat" are strongly related to low body cognitions, whereas another study indicates that believing oneself to be "too fat" is not necessarily related to low body satisfaction for black women. Some studies with African American participants have indicated distinct experiences of the body and the meanings of beauty. The families and communities of the African American participants supported their appearance and style, and also appreciated a fuller physique than did European American participant families and communities. The positive feedback that the African American participants receive from their immediate family and community was theorized to have a positive influence on their self-esteem. The African American participants also reported having a stronger support group among their peers than the European American participants did. Although the European American adolescents reported dieting as a strategy to establish group affiliation with others, they also reported comparing themselves with other girls and consequently feeling negative about themselves and other girls. This act of comparing fostered a sense of competition among these participants.

Conversely, the African American participants reported having very supportive relationships with others and their affiliations were not based on comparisons and competition. I can remember when I was in my early twenties; I was working in the Human Resource Department at a major bank. The department had just undergone some major consolidation changes, which brought several other departments together to work in one room. The department hired several workers from a temporary employment agency. One day at the lunch room, one of the female temp workers came up to me and said that I was so skinny and that I was the first black woman that she had met that did not have a big butt. I couldn't believe that she had said this to me and in front of other employees. I was startled for a moment, and then I looked at her and told her that not all black women have big butts. The second time I experienced another stereotype about my body was when I was in my late thirties and I was working as a Human Resource Recruiter at a credit union. I had just finished an interview with an Asian male and I was walking him to the front door. This man looked at me and said, "You're so thin! How do you do it? Do you diet?" I answered him and said that I do not diet. I just merely stay active and watch what I eat.

He said "Wow!" I can't believe it." He also said that most African American people that he had seen were very big. I told him that no matter what a person's ethnicity was, they come in all different shapes and sizes. He was very surprised to see how small in size I was. I was very surprised at how people of other cultures and ethnicities view African American women in terms of body size. The stereotype categorized African American women as all being the same. By bringing up this situation, I am reminded that there have been many studies over the years to support the fact that the United States is now reporting a weight epidemic among most Americans. In some of the more recent studies, the findings show that over 50 percent of most Americans are overweight, and the statistics show that these numbers are steadily increasing each year. In the dominant white American discourse, the body is judged on the basis of a person's physical weight and appearance. Within white American culture, attractiveness is sometimes linked to virtue, goodness, kindness, and nurturance, and thinness has been associated with self-control. For example; if one is skinny, one is perceived to have taken action, if one is not, or is overweight, then one is perceived as lazy and inactive. Unfortunately, in today's society these images seem to be increasing especially with models on television, movies, magazines, and catalogs. The most important aspect to remember is to accept your body and weight in terms of who you are.

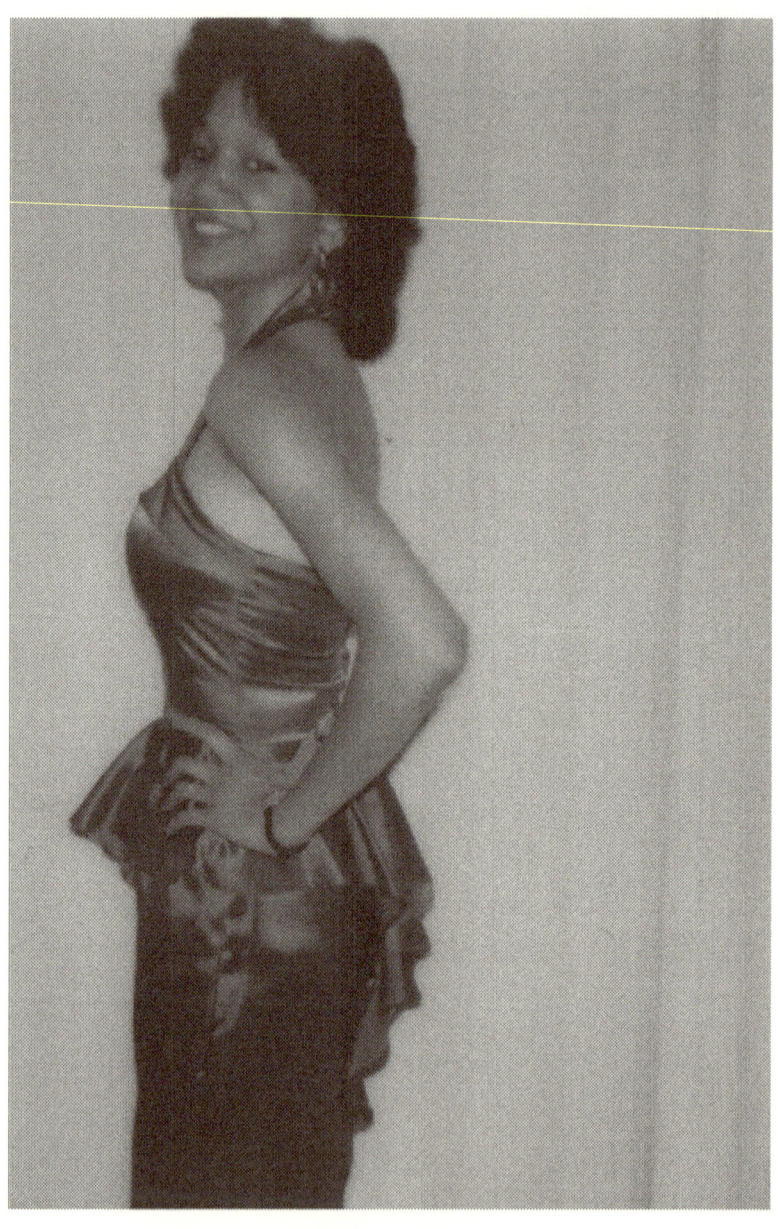

My 21ˢᵗ Birthday

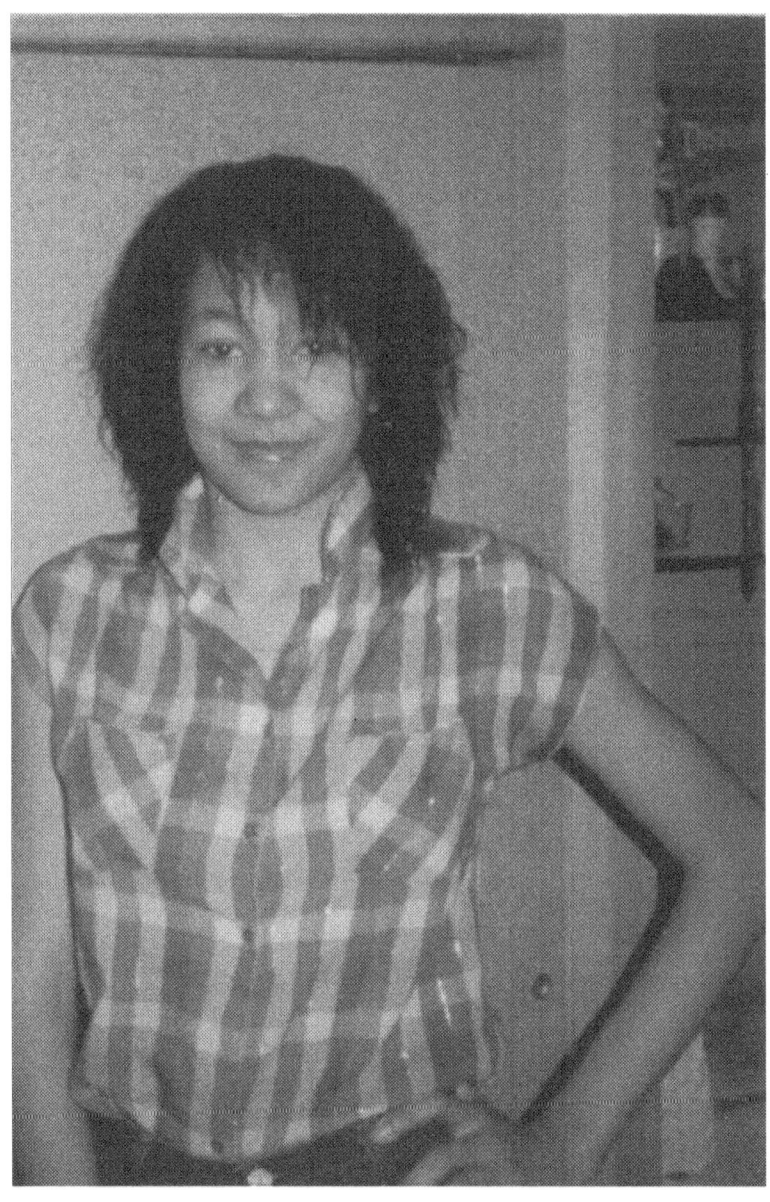

Me as a teenager

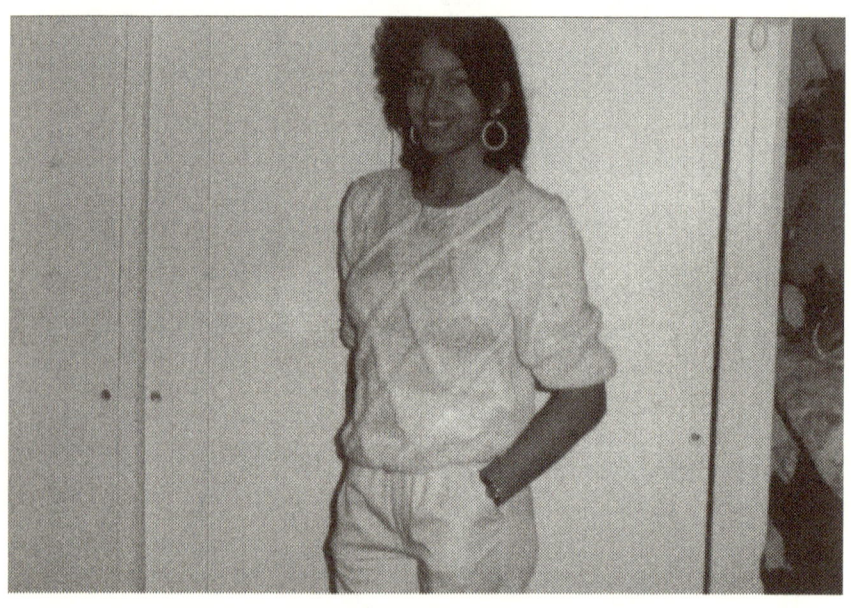

Me in my early twenties

CHAPTER 6

What Exercises Work?
Fitness for Children and Inactive Seniors; and Choosing the Right
Fitness Equipment

Kids exercise all the time without even thinking about it. They are just being active, like when they run around outside or play kickball at school, which is a great form of exercise. What else counts as exercise? Playing sports, dancing, doing push-ups, and even reaching down to touch your toes. Exercise strengthens muscles. The following are some exercises and activities that build strong muscles: push-ups, pull-ups, tug-of-war, rowing, running, in-line skating, and bike riding. Most kids are pretty flexible, which means that they can bend and stretch their bodies without much trouble. Being flexible means having a full range of motion, being able to move your arms and legs freely, without feeling tightness or pain. Things that help with flexibility are tumbling, gymnastics, yoga, dancing (especially ballet), martial arts, and simple stretches such as touching your toes or side stretches. What can families do to help children create healthy habits? The family is the primary influence on a child's habits. All adult family members should become educated, involved, and committed to setting the right examples for the children in their family. Everything you do at home affects the habits of your kid's development, from the vocabulary you use, to the foods you bring home, to the examples you set with your own eating habits and physical activity.

Tip #40: Learn to read food labels.

An excellent tip is to read the labels on the food you buy. This can give you lots of information. When you buy heart-healthy foods, it helps to break the bad snacking habit. Get the kids involved with label reading and make shopping a healthy game.

Tip #41: Purchase heart-healthy books and get involved in programs just for kids. The American Heart Association already has some programs to help kids lead heart-healthy lives. Look into programs such as Jump Rope for Heart, Hoops for Heart, and Heart Power.

Overweight children are more likely to be overweight adults. Successfully preventing or treating obesity in childhood may help reduce the risk of heart disease and other complications. When my son spends the day at his grandparents' house, he keeps my parents very busy. He likes to go outside and have his grandparents participate in many activities with him. My parents, on the other hand, are also very active people, even though they like to watch a lot of television. Sometimes too much TV can cut into a person's workout time. Fitness, however, doesn't mean that you have to give up your favorite shows. A person can work out in front of the television. It is absolutely possible to improve your fitness level in front of the TV if the intensity is adequate. Studies show that American men average twenty-nine hours a week of TV watching.

Women generally watch up to about thirty-four hours of television. That gives us a lot of time to fit in some extra activity. Most people can fit in fitness workouts during commercials. This can be a good option for beginners and seniors. Some of the exercises to do include push-ups. If the floor push-ups are too difficult for you, start off by standing up with your hands on the wall, then pushing back; do this ten times, increasing the reps as the exercise gets easier. For chair squats; stand up, sit down—but not all the way!—then push yourself back up again. Do this for the length of one commercial. As it gets easier, do it again for the next commercial. March in place. Move both your arms and legs; and add jumping jacks to increase the intensity. You can also use resistance tubing, dumbbells or even books or cans of soup: Do upper body exercises while seated on a chair. Examples are bicep curls, overhead shoulder presses, side arm raises, front arm raises, and tricep extensions. Other exercises include lying on the floor; do side-lying leg raises for the outer hip and inner thigh, with or without weights, sitting up on the floor, use resistance bands to do seated rows. Pretend you're rowing a boat. To get the most out of your TV workout, do something different every day, and remember to do the things you like to do.

Older adults age sixty-five and older can also get health benefits from exercise. Even patients with chronic illnesses such as heart disease, high blood pressure, diabetes, and arthritis can exercise safely. Many of these conditions are improved with exercise. If you are not sure if exercise is safe for you or if you are currently inactive, ask your doctor. Exercise, however, is only good for you if you are feeling well.

> **Tip #42: Wait to exercise until you feel better, if you have a cold, flu, or other illness. If you miss exercise for more than two weeks, be sure to start slowly again. You should call your doctor if your muscles or joints are sore the next day after exercising; you may have done too much. Next time, exercise at a lower intensity. If the pain or discomfort persists, you should talk to your doctor. You should also talk to your doctor if you have any of the following symptoms while exercising: chest pain or pressure, trouble breathing or fatigue, excessive shortness of breath, lightheadedness or dizziness, difficulty with balance or not seeing.**

Exercising does not have to be expensive, even though it may be tough to fit it into a busy day. You can create an affordable home gym. Your home gym can be as lavish as you like, with the mega-machines and expensive cardio equipment, or as simple as a good pair of athletic shoes.

For the budget minded, a home gym doesn't have to cost a thing. When I first started working out, I was in high school. My older brother and I pooled our money to purchase a workout bench. It was around forty dollars, and that seemed like a lot of money. We put the workout bench on our backyard patio and used it every day. It allowed only for leg lifts and bench presses. Eventually, we started using it only occasionally, and then we stopped using the bench altogether. What I didn't know was that I could have made my own set of weights without spending an extra dime.

The nice thing about weight training is that anything with weights will work as a dumbbell; a full water bottle or a bag full of sand. Your body doesn't know the difference. Whether you're out-fitting a home gym or traveling, there are a variety of things you can use as a dumbbell, such as full soup cans; these are great for lighter weights. Some larger cans weigh up to a pound or more and can be used for upper body exercises. Full water bottles, such as a large water bottle holding around 33.8 fluid ounces, can give you a little more than two pounds when full of water. Fill it with sand, rocks, or loose change (a good way to put pennies to use!), and you'll get even more weight.

Save your old milk jugs and fill them with sand, loose change, or water for weights with ready-made handles. PVC pipes can also be used as dumbbells. You can fill them with sand and tape off the ends with duct tape to avoid spillage. This is a great idea, since PVC pipes come in all shapes and sizes, and many of them fit perfectly in your hand. You can also fill tennis balls and tennis cans with sand and or loose change for some great handheld weights. Most of these materials can be found around your house or at your local hardware store. If you're not into making weights yourself, there are some other alternatives for finding cheap equipment. If you don't mind a little bargain hunting, you can find cheap exercise equipment in a variety of places, such as garage sales. I almost always see exercise gear at garage sales, and some of it's even worth buying. Pick up the newspaper to find weekend garage sales in your area. I believe that you will find something. The retail chain called "Play It Again Sports" buys and sells new and used exercise equipment. If you have one in your area, it's worth checking out, especially for their dumbbell selection, which is usually pretty good. Major discount retail stores have very competitive prices, especially when it comes to exercise equipment.

They have a great selection of hex weights that are reasonably priced. They also carry resistance bands, which are another cheap alternative to buying weights. Ebay, internet and classified ads are other good sources. People are always selling and buying things, especially exercise equipment they never use. Check out your newspaper or the Internet; you can often find some great deals.

When I was approximately nineteen years old, I went with my older sister to Holiday Health Spa. We had a free day pass to use the facility and the equipment. They had a full-service state-of-the-art fitness facility. The sales staff talked us into joining and signing up for membership. At first, we were very excited and were using the facility every week. Eventually, we started going less and less frequently, until eventually we stopped going altogether. This was unfortunate, because we had signed a one-year contract, and we were paying for something that we weren't really using. This was a lesson that I learned early in life. Never sign up for something that you are not 100 percent committed to, especially when you're a young adult or adolescent on a tight budget.

Adolescence is a time when girls begin to mature into women, and they are very vulnerable. They take into consideration their body, and they try all sorts of exercise and diet tips. Girls start developing breasts and hips, and their hormones go into overdrive, causing hair and skin blemishes. And this is also when menstruation usually begins. There is no standard starting age for adolescents; it can start when a girl is as young as nine or when she is well into her teens.

Adolescence is also a perfect time in life to develop good exercise habits. When a girl's body begins producing the hormone estrogen, which helps trigger sexual development, she may notice an increase in body fat. She may then try a variety of crash diets to maintain what she thinks is an ideal body image. Physical therapists agree that exercise is a safer way to maintain ideal body weight than by dieting itself. Such therapists can help the adolescent girl determine her appropriate body weight and encourage her to enjoy aerobic and resistance exercise, such as walking, swimming, or dancing.

Giving birth and raising a family can also be the most exciting times of your life. But you may be so busy focusing on the child that's growing inside you that you neglect the changing needs of your own body. When you're pregnant, your posture, center of gravity, and body size all change as the fetus develops. Keep mind that all these changes might be accompanied by some discomfort. A physical therapist can determine what's causing your pain and can tell you if it's pregnancy related. A physical therapist will start off with a complete evaluation to determine how your body movements might be causing added strain on your spine. You'll learn how to maintain good posture throughout the day, and even at night while you're sleeping.

Even if you're not especially athletic, it's important that both you and your baby are in the best shape possible during your pregnancy. Physical therapists recommend some guidelines on safe exercise for expectant mothers. These guidelines take into account the safety of the fetus and encourage regular exercise—not rigorous, competitive exercise. A complete exercise program includes flexibility, low-impact aerobics, muscle strengthening, endurance, and relaxation exercises. Key muscle groups targeted during prenatal exercise include the postural muscles— along the spine and between the shoulder blades, the abdominal muscles, and iliopsoas (the deep muscle in front of the pelvis and spine), and the pelvic floor muscles: It is that layer of deep muscle within the pelvis which is a base of support for the pelvic organs and opening from the vagina, urethra, and rectum. When I was pregnant with my son, I made sure that I stayed very active. Proper nutrition was also very important during pregnancy, as well as exercise. Because I maintained such a slim figure over the years, I didn't show my pregnancy shape until I was approximately six months along into my pregnancy; meaning I was able to wear regular clothes until I was six months into my pregnancy. That was when and I had to start wearing maternity clothes. In fact, many of my coworkers didn't even believe that I was six months along in my pregnancy until I showed them the shape of my belly. When I was in the hospital, being prepped for my C-section, the nurse lifted up my gown on the table and said, "How cute, it looks like a basketball."

After you've had your baby, you'll want to get back on track with postnatal exercise. Your physical therapists can evaluate you for postural problems or abdominal weakness and can then put you on a program to gradually strengthen those muscles. The program may include pelvic floor exercises to prevent incontinence, or difficulty with bladder control. Simple attention to little details in everyday life will make a big difference in your comfortable recovery. Your baby's changing table, for instance, should be at waist level, so you don't have to bend forward or strain your back. In fact, try to keep from bending over from the waist as much as possible. If you stand a lot, try resting one foot on a stool or box. This will give your back added support. Lots of touching, holding, and interacting is good for your baby and you too. When picking up your baby or younger child, remember to protect your spine. Bend your knees, keep the child close to your body, and lift with your leg muscles, not your back. Also, don't carry your baby all day on one hip. During this time of learning about handling your baby correctly and gently, you need to remember to be careful not to do your own body any damage.

CHAPTER 7

Jealousy Rears Its Ugly Head!
Dealing with the Comments and Criticism (Body Envy)

When you head to the gym or even out to a party, how do you react when you see someone that you feel is thinner or better looking than you? Does that twinge of jealousy shoot up your spine? Or do you think, "Wow, they look great! Good for them!" If you're like most, chances are your first reaction may be to escort them to the nearest all-you-can-eat buffet. So what's your diagnosis? Are you a mean or insanely jealous person? Don't fret, it's just a small case of body envy—we've all had it. Just remember, your body is beautiful no matter what shape or size it is, and jealousy only tears down your self-esteem. At the moment, body image, mentioned earlier, is a larger deal with the female population than with the male. However, it is very important for you to know that the male gender is rapidly becoming more and more aware of their bodies and how they look, and so many men are jealous of what they see in the media and in others, much like women. The answer is that as long as there has been human life, there has been the acknowledgment of body image, jealousy, competition, and all other things that lead to men and women of all ages trying to battle against the body image struggle. We all know the feeling of not living up to our usual potential in some way or receiving a comment from a friend or loved one that just makes you want to beat yourself up.

A survey of college students found that they would prefer to marry an embezzler, drug user, shoplifter, or blind person than someone who is overweight. Fifty percent of women between the ages of eighteen and twenty-five would rather be run over by a truck than to be fat. No wonder why people are becoming ill with life-threatening diseases. In a new age of medical technology, processes like plastic surgery and "tummy tucks" can give you back your confidence by making you more attractive (or so they say), at a high price physically, mentally, and dollar-wise. Not only are people going through supplement pills and other drugs to get skinny again, but women in today's society are focusing on breast enlargement, while younger men are more often abusing steroids in order to get bulkier. Today, I get compliments from people who admire my size and want to know my secret for staying thin. I also get cynical remarks from co-workers who will look at me and say, "You're so skinny, you make me sick." I have been called names in the past such as skinny Minnie, and Olive Oil. I have been given serious glaring looks with envy that could kill.

Most of these comments were coming from my co-workers who were supposed to be older, more mature, professional women. But this type of jealousy is also becoming more apparent in children as well. It is evident that parents also have to watch their children and teach them from a young age not to get persuaded by the media or market when it comes to having an ideal body image. Kids must be taught that both the media and the market can be useful and fun, but overall they should learn to be happy with who they are and to have pride in not only what they look like but, most importantly, what they can do. The youth of today's society also forget that a good relationship doesn't dwell on the fact of only appearance; instead it relies on a mental connection between partners which is forever more pleasing and pleasurable. A person who doesn't have a strong self-image may feel that he or she is not getting his or her "fair share" and that others always "get the breaks." All emotions, even jealousy, are trying to tell us something about ourselves. Jealousy is a fear of losing power. When we find out what we're missing, that fear goes away. Acknowledging our jealousy is the first step in overcoming it.

If we're ashamed of feeling jealous, we may try to mask it with "protective emotions" such as anger, frustration, or resentment. Typically we're jealous of things we want, not of things we need.

Tip #43: **Ask yourself how you can work toward what you want, and make a list of all that you do have that you feel good about.**

Tip #44: **Confront your jealousy head on. Once you let go of any standards you are using to psychologically imprison yourself, you are free to appreciate other people's good fortune without thinking you're not enough. Not everything in life is equal or fair, but to be dishonest about your own feelings is wrong.**

Tip #45: **Express interest in what is important to other people, and then you can share, honestly, what is important to you. Remember, there will always be someone out there who is more beautiful, more talented, and more successful. But so what?**

Nothing is wrong with wanting to look good. Everyone should be able to wear what they think looks good, although sometimes instruments like the media put a different perspective on what really looks good and what really makes money. When people see someone that is naturally gorgeous and has money and leads a life that is all play and no work, they may tend to try to look and act like that person. They become crazed with new fashion trends that are built around this popular star or icon; however, some take it to the next level. Some people are just not able to pull off the "hot" new look, and this upsets them. Soon they begin to rationalize, and thus bad eating habits emerge.

When it comes to males, they seem to want to become larger and more muscular; however, the problems that come from wanting to be this way are often very serious. Many young men who try to improve their body size and shape use a drug called steroids. As well as being illegal, steroids are bad for your body over a long period of time and they are also addictive. An increasing number of adolescents are turning to steroids for cosmetic reasons. They come from cities and rural areas, from poor families and wealthy ones. They are of all races and nationalities. The common link among them is the desire to look good and to perform and feel better at almost any cost. Steroid users, especially the young, are apt to ignore or deny warnings about health risks. If they see their friends growing taller and stronger on steroids, then they also want the same benefits. Steroids can become addictive, and some users continue to take these drugs in spite of physical problems, negative affects on relationships, or nervousness and irritability. They also spend large amounts of time and money obtaining these drugs and experience withdrawal symptoms such as mood swings, fatigue, restlessness, loss of appetite, insomnia, reduced sex drive, and the desire to take more steroids. The most dangerous of the withdrawal symptom is depression, because it sometimes can lead to suicide attempts.

So your best friend wears a size zero and complains that it's too big on her! Jealous? Who wouldn't be? Sure, there are times when everyone else seems to have more, do more, or look better. But is that really the case? Jealousy may reflect a person's view of him or herself. It's more about how people feel about themselves and whether they're confident about who they are. For many, jealousy has to do with their personal relationships. You might become jealous, for example, if you feel that your partner is not paying enough attention to you. Jealousy also may be provoked if your partner or spouse consistently makes you feel uncomfortable through both their words and their actions. With this in mind, a person can develop negative self-esteem or rebellion, and this can motivate the individual into bad eating habits or depression. In any relationship, trust and mutual respect are essential to keep the relationship flourishing and keeping the communication strong. A person who has a poor self-image may feel threatened and believe that she has nothing to offer to keep someone else interested. Most jealousy arises when someone feels insecure and threatened either by loss of the relationship or by someone else getting the attention she craves. When you handle jealousy properly, though, it doesn't have to be a disaster.

Tip #46: **Know your strengths. What do you specifically bring to the table? Don't compare yourself with anyone else, because then you're only sabotaging your own uniqueness.**

Tip #47: **Affirm the other person. Today is his or her turn to shine, tomorrow it will be yours. Use jealousy to emulate the object of your jealousy and fuel you to accomplish your goals and grow. If he or she can do it, so can you.**

Tip #48: **If someone else is toxic to you, because he or she is constantly bragging just to make you feel jealous, then change the subject, or if need be, simply remove yourself from that person's presence; if necessary, permanently!**

Years ago, when my mother was working for the college district, her office co-workers were primarily female. She told me that they used to make comments in regard to her size. She told me that they used to say, "Barbara, you are so skinny," when in actuality, she had put on a little weight in her middle-age years, so her weight was in proportion to her height. Unfortunately, the women in her office were overweight and were jealous of her size. In a way, they envied her and wanted to be more like her physically. They did not know how to develop a friendship with my mother and approach her, to find out what her methods to maintaining her weight were and how she was satisfied with her body size and shape.

Overcoming jealousy is easier said than done! Whether it is a conscious word or thought in the back of your mind, jealousy is something we all struggle with daily. Sometimes those little thoughts that creep into our minds don't sound like jealousy, but they are. Overcoming jealousy is a constant challenge. However, I know firsthand that when jealousy is not overcome, it leads to bitterness. In fact, the Bible even addresses jealousy. James 3:16 says, "For where jealousy and selfish ambition exist, there is disorder in every evil thing." From this wisdom, we learn that wrong thinking produces wrong living. When we have thoughts of jealousy or feelings of envy, our lives will be characterized by confusion, disorder, and feelings of worthlessness. No good actions will come from an evil and jealous spirit. Dealing with jealousy is essential. When uncontrolled jealousy and envy are intense and unrelenting, you may need to seek professional counseling or even see a doctor.

Tip #49: Call your local mental health clinic, employee counseling service, or therapist if:

1. Jealousy or envy is interfering with important relationships in your life.

2. You are so distracted by feelings of envy and jealousy that you can't focus on things that you want to accomplish.

3. You have been consumed with jealousy and envy most of your life.

4. You find yourself blaming or threatening people of whom you are jealous or envious.

5. You avoid venturing out because you are afraid that you'll see things that make you envious or jealous.

Acknowledge your feelings. Denying your feelings is stressful. Admit to yourself that you're jealous and learn from it. Interestingly, women seem to find it easier to acknowledge jealousy than men do. Ask yourself why you're jealous. Question your assumptions. Turn envy into admiration. If you envy someone because she has some quality, such as being slim, slender, and fit, then take steps to cultivate that quality that you admire.

Another method for treating jealousy is through hypnotherapy. This is just the art of using hypnosis as therapy to treat the issue of many problems, including jealousy, overeating, dieting, etc. It is used to help people make useful changes in their thoughts and their behaviors. Therapists work very closely with people to train their minds to learn to be able to become more flexible in their thinking; to help them stop engaging in unwanted automated thinking, feelings, and behavior; and, most importantly, to help them aim themselves in a more useful direction.

The approach, therefore, is to tackle the unwanted thinking and behavior head on, rather than the more common practice of spending hours going over the past looking for some hidden meaning, in the hopes that discovering and coming to terms with such will magically transform everything. Useful rapid results can very often be achieved by using hypnotherapy without resorting to going over the past. Hypnotherapy is a process whereby you become deeply or lightly relaxed, guided by words, phrases, suggestions, and imagination. Hypnotherapy is often one of the more important ways that therapists use to work with clients to help them. There are also, as indicated, numerous techniques that can be used, from direct and indirect suggestion to indirect use of metaphor.

Most techniques have proven useful, though some people respond better than others. Therapists tend to blend them to do their best to ensure rapid, positive results. The unconscious mind is immensely powerful and very capable of change. With hypnotherapy, your unconscious mind becomes very responsive to all highly productive and beneficial ideas and suggestions when they are delivered well, and you essentially become re-educated at a deeper level.

CHAPTER 8

See Your Doctor Regularly!
Being Underweight or Overweight and Maintaining Proper Health

Annual medical exams are important to help people of all ages maintain good health, by spotting potential problems in their early stages. At each visit, a doctor will usually make the routine checks of functions like your heart, lungs, and blood pressure. As you reach adulthood, a cholesterol test may be given. Because cholesterol deposits start forming early in life, it's not a bad idea to start testing your cholesterol as early as age twenty, perhaps sooner if you have a strong family history of heart disease. In addition, a doctor may suggest a complete blood analysis every few years, in which levels of iron, glucose, uric acid, hemoglobin, and many other substances are measured. By age forty, it is recommended that women have an annual mammogram and Pap smear, in addition to their regular medical exam. Meanwhile, men over forty should receive a test for prostate cancer during their yearly physical. To find out more about annual checkups, contact a doctor in your area. You should consider your doctor as your partner in health care. As a partner, there are things you can do to enable her to provide the best care for you. One of the first things you can, and should, do is have questions ready, so that when you're choosing a new physician, you'll know that you'll be picking the best one for you.

First of all, if you don't have a doctor you see on a regular basis, make it a priority to find one. When you have a doctor, stick with her and see her regularly, instead of going to different ones. Everytime you are sick, she will become more familiar with you and your history, allowing you to establish a trusting, long-term relationship. If you choose a family practitioner, he or she can take care of all of your general illnesses and health care needs. If your illness is more severe or you are more comfortable with someone with more experience treating specific illnesses, you might choose a physician who is a specialist. The best way to find a doctor is through word of mouth, asking friends, coworkers, and acquaintances if they can recommend someone. Schedule an appointment to meet the doctor before you are sick. This will give you a chance to decide whether or not you are comfortable with meeting and making her your regular doctor. To properly treat you, a doctor must know the details of your health history and health practices. If you are uncomfortable sharing your past sexual history, your smoking, diet, exercise habits, or mental health issues like depression; your doctor cannot properly assess your health, order necessary tests, or prescribe correct medication.

When I became pregnant with my son, I researched several hospitals, including one of the major franchise hospitals in Southern California. I drove around the corner to view the outside appearance of the building. I even went into the maternity ward to get a look at the inside appearance and interaction of the staff. I selected my doctor by looking up his credentials in the physician's directory. So it is very important to do your research before you see your doctor. During your get-acquainted appointment, talk with a doctor about issues that are important to you. The importance of seeing a doctor regularly is significant, because the Centers for Disease Control and Prevention (the CDC) has referred to the problem of obesity in the United States as a public health epidemic, and research indicates that the situation continues to grow. Seeing a doctor regularly is very important because she can explain about being overweight and what obesity means to you.

Doctors can also make you aware if you weigh too much or too little for your height. They can determine if you really are too fat or too thin and can monitor your weight to see if you have entered a danger zone which can lead to health problems. The following basic definitions are designed to explain healthy and unhealthy weight. **Body composition** is the makeup of lean body mass and body fat in the body. **Lean body mass** refers to your arms, legs, back, neck, and abdomen muscles. It also includes your heart muscle and the tissues of your internal organs, as well as water and bone. The lean body mass is the part of your body you want to preserve or expand. The quantity of lean body mass you have is the most important factor in determining the metabolic rate at which you burn calories. The greater your lean body mass, the higher your metabolic rate and the more calories you will burn while sitting or lying down. A higher metabolic rate makes it easier to maintain your weight. A regular program of strength training and resistance training can increase the amount and the strength of your muscles. This in turn will also increase your metabolic rate. Body fat is one of the basic components that make up the body structure. Body fat has many important functions, including acting as a storage site for energy, which it issues when your body is inactive or in times of illness or injury.

Body fat is also important because it protects your organs from injury and insulates your body, by keeping it warm. There are two categories of body fat: central fat and storage fat. Central fat is necessary for normal, healthy functioning. It is stored in small amounts in your bone marrow, organs, central nervous system, and muscles. In men, central fat is roughly 3 percent of body weight. In women, the percentage of central fat is about 12 percent. This higher percentage takes into account some sex-specific facts believed to be critical for normal reproductive function found in breasts, pelvis, hips, and thighs. Storage fat is the other type of body fat. It accumulates beneath the skin, in certain specific areas inside your body, and in your muscles. It also includes the deep fat that protects your internal organs from injury.

Men and women have similar amounts of storage fat. Storage fat increases when you gain weight. It is what you want to lose when you lose weight. Everyone requires a certain amount of body fat. It is desirable to have some storage fat, due to the protective role it plays in your body, but most is considered expendable. Too much or too little storage of fat is unhealthy and may lead to serious health risks. What is the healthy range of body fat? Ranges differ for men and women depending on their age.

For the average adult, the healthy range of body fat from ages eighteen to thirty-nine is 21–32 percent for females, and 18–19 percent for males. For ages forty to fifty-nine, it is 23–33 percent for females, and 11–21 percent for males. For ages sixty-two to seventy-nine, it is 24–35 percent for females and 12–24 percent for males. Professional and superior amateur athletes, however, often have a body fat percentage much lower than the average person. Body fat has been as low as 3.3 percent in male marathon runners and as low as 14.5 percent in female Olympic swimmers. Overweight and obese individuals, unfortunately, have too much body fat, increasing their risk for many diseases. To most people, obesity means being very overweight. However, there is a distinction between the terms "overweight" and "obese" which has to do with the differences in body weight. An *overweight* person has a body mass index (BMI) of 25 to 29.99 percent, or is between twenty-five to thirty pounds over the recommended weight for the person's height. *Obesity* is the condition of being considerably overweight and refers to a person with a BMI of 30 or greater or who is at least thirty pounds over the recommended weight for a person's height.

An important note: Muscular athletes and bodybuilders can be overweight without being obese. Cases of obesity happen when a person consumes more calories than he or she burns. Reasons for this imbalance include genetic, environmental, psychological, and other factors.

Genetic factors of obesity tend to run in families, suggesting a genetic cause.

Yet families who share diet and lifestyle habits may also contribute to obesity. Separating obese from genetic factors is often difficult. Even so, science shows that heredity is linked to obesity. Environmental factors may also strongly influence obesity. This includes lifestyle habits such as diet and level of physical activity. American culture tends to eat high-fat foods and put taste and convenience before nutrition, and most Americans do not get enough physical activity. Regarding psychological factors, many people eat in response to negative emotions such as boredom, sadness, or anger. Most overweight people have no more psychological problems than people of average weight. However, up to 10 percent of mildly obese people trying to lose weight have an eating disorder. This disorder is even more common in people who are severely obese. During a binge eating episode, people feel they cannot control how much they are eating and eat large amounts of food. Those with the most severe binge eating problems are also likely to have symptoms of depression and low self-esteem. These people may have more difficulty losing weight and keeping it off than people without binge-eating problems.

Other factors and some illnesses can lead to obesity or a tendency to gain weight, develop problems with thyroids, Cushing's syndrome, depression, and certain neurological problems. Drugs such as steroids and some antidepressants may also cause weight problems. Your doctor can tell you if underlying medical conditions are causing the weight gain or making the weight loss difficult. Who can become overweight or obese? Just about anyone is at risk for being overweight—this includes men, women, and children of all ages and races. Some people, however, are at greater risk than others.

Other studies have shown that obesity is especially prevalent among women with lower incomes and is more common among African American and Mexican American women than among white women. Among African Americans, the proportion of women who are obese is 80 percent higher than the proportion of African American men who are obese. This gender difference also is seen among Mexican American women and men, but the percentage of white non-Hispanic men and women who are obese is about the same. What happens when you gain weight? Fully grown adults gain both lean body mass and storage fat when they gain weight. The amount of fat gained usually far exceeds the amount of lean body mass gained: about 60 to 80 percent fat and 20 to 40 percent lean body mass. For instance, if you gain ten pounds, about six to eight pounds should be fat and two to four pounds would be lean body mass.

This would mean increases not only in your fat tissue, but also in your muscles, stomach, intestines and other organs, bowels, and water. These percentages would vary if you were involved in a training program specifically aimed at increasing muscle mass. What happens when you lose weight? You lose water, lean body mass, and storage fat. From a health standpoint, and to maintain your metabolic rate, it is better to preserve as much lean body mass as possible while you reduce your body fat. How much fat and lean body mass should you lose when you lose weight? Experts have determined that during the early weeks of weight loss, at least 75 percent of the weight you lose should be fat loss and not more than 25 percent should come from lean body mass. As you continue to lose weight, especially if certain types of exercises are included in your weight loss plan, fat loss should be about 90 percent of the weight you lose, and lean body mass should be about 10 percent. Weight management is an important part of everyone's life. It is essential, especially for individuals to continue to sustain a healthy lifestyle.

It is also important to get regular medical care from your doctor. By working with your doctor, you can prevent health problems or find them early. It's important to feel comfortable with your doctor, so you can talk about any health issue. If you don't have a regular doctor, get one through your health plan. Many families qualify for free or low-cost health insurance through Medicaid or income qualifying medical plans. People without health coverage do not have to go without good medical care. You can contact your local city or county offices or any public or community health clinic to get a doctor. One should establish a routine of regular checkups. By so doing, you'll have the opportunity to develop a relationship with your doctor.

Tip #50: Ask questions. Keep track of potential questions and a list of any unusual symptoms you may have experienced. A notebook, small enough to carry in your purse or pocket, is good for this purpose. Keep this notebook handy, when you're in the doctor's office, whether for a regular checkup or for an illness, so you can rely on your notes rather than your memory to update your doctor on any new symptoms you're experiencing. Ask your doctor which signs and symptoms warrant an office visit and which might require just a phone call, or if it's OK to wait for a day or two to see if they self-correct.

Tip #51: Keep a list of all medications, vitamins, and supplements you take. This is an important step in remembering any potential adverse interactions with new medications prescribed by your doctor.

CHAPTER 9

Colors, Styles, and Patterns That Will Make You Look Smaller!
Myths and Misconceptions About Fashion

Improve your fashion and skills with these simple tips to enhance your shape and make your wardrobe work for you. The clothing you select will impact your physical appearance, and also how you are perceived by others. Everybody has body imperfections. The following tips are for individuals who can accept their imperfections, but at the same time also would like to de-emphasize these imperfections. An important note to remember is to have very good posture and always stand up straight and to carry yourself gracefully. This will give you the appearance of looking taller and sets off a look of self-confidence.

Tip #52: Be familiar with your body and what looks good on it. Normally, a person is attracted to clothing and colors that will flatter her figure. Use past experience to your advantage and rely on your own intuition—sometimes fashion and beauty come naturally. Feel free to experiment. Watch out for those skinny mirrors in department stores that can be somewhat misleading. If a style didn't look good on you in the past, it won't look good now; unless you have made some significant changes to your figure.

Tip #53: Have your clothes tailored. Tailored clothes flatter most figures.

Tip #54: Purchase similar pieces of the clothes you already have that you feel will flatter your figure.

Tip #55: Shoulder pads will help you balance large breasts and wide hips but keep them slim.

Tip #56: Try dressing monochromatic, all one color for a slimmer look, then accentuate the look with a sleek scarf.

Teenagers often use hairstyles, jewelry, trendy, and funky clothing to set themselves apart from the crowd, and at the same time fit in. For a teenage girl, fashion plays an important part in self-esteem and identity. Styles are always changing, and as teens grow up, they find out just how far they are willing to go to make their mark on the world. Some hairstyles and clothing trends that were once considered taboo are now acceptable; as teens discover who they are and what they want to represent. If you're a teen, you can discover what's hot in teen fashions and accessories by going to local malls and department stores.

Fashion advice for vintage clothes shopping: Why would anyone want to wear vintage clothing? First of all, it's fun. When you wear vintage, you stand out from the crowd. The chances of someone also wearing the same exact outfit to that special event are slim and none.

More and more high school girls are shopping vintage for dances and proms because it guarantees originality. Vintage clothing is also nostalgic. For the thrifty, the prices on vintage items should be incentive enough. Local thrift stores, flea markets, and yard sales are excellent sources of old clothing at unbelievable prices. Broke? Go volunteer to help clean out Grandma's closet. Vintage clothing can be teamed up with modern apparel or mixed and matched with other vintage pieces. This also includes plus size fashions for large women. Just because you're a large woman doesn't mean you have to wear the boring ultra-drab clothing that's commonly available. In America, the average dress size is going up, and there are an increasing number of women who want to look naturally bold and chic; and fortunately, designers are listening to consumers and are creating attractive, plus-size fashions for women.

Unless you know exactly what to look for, shopping for clothing can be frustrating and time-consuming. Spending your money wisely, and finding fashions that flatter your figure and skin tone is not impossible. Choose clothes that fit. Don't buy loose clothing that hangs on your frame. This will add bulk and make you appear larger.

On the other hand, stay away from clothes that will fit perfectly if you lose five to ten pounds. Clingy fabrics are unforgiving and will show every flaw and bulge. Buy clothes that you are comfortable in, standing up and sitting down. Wear proper undergarments. Always wear bras and panties that fit you well. Bras that ride up your back will not enhance your bust and you will probably experience unwanted bulges. Consider investing in a body shaper to look sleek in a suit or dress. Many tanks and halter tops now have built-in bras.

Too much white makes you look larger, so limit this color. Don't even think about wearing white slacks or pantyhose, unless you want to add bulk. Top off your look with accessories that match your style. Choose a mid-length necklace. Short-hanging necklaces and chokers tend to make your neck appear larger. Don't over-accessorize.

How to choose the best jeans for your figure? Don't buy jeans because the size on the label looks good. Sizes and cuts vary widely by the brand, so start with your general size range and don't be reluctant to choose a size larger than what you usually wear. Choose a comfortable pair of jeans that will fit well and will look best on you.

The darker the color, the better. If you're concerned about extra weight, stay away from light-colored or stonewashed jeans. Dark indigo blue and black denim jeans with an added Lycra will make you look slimmer and will go with just about anything. Choose angled back pockets to help minimize your backside, and stay away from jeans that have no pockets and all.

Tip #57: Look for a long hem. When you go shopping, wear a pair of shoes with heels that are at least similar to what you usually wear with jeans. For thinner-looking legs, the hem of the jeans should cover a good part of your shoes and almost reach the floor. Keep in mind that jeans shrink, so when you go shopping, it's better to go with the longer pair.

Tip #58: Go with the boot cut. Stay away from large flare legs, which will add bulk. Boot-cut jeans have just the right amount of curve at the bottom of the legs to look stylish and make your legs appear longer. Look for colors that make a fashion statement. Women are generally drawn to colors that flatter their figure and complexion. Your favorite color shouldn't always appear in your wardrobe if it doesn't do a thing for you. If you are in the majority, the color you want most often to wear matches the image you want to reflect and is the color that makes you look and feel good.

What does the color of your clothing say about you? Black says conservative yet sexy, and you know that black is versatile. Wearing black clothing makes you appear thinner, giving your self-esteem a turbo boost. Pink is traditional and charming. Pink is feminine all the way. A pink and black combo is a trendy way for women to add a mature color to their otherwise girly image.

Red is bold and vibrant: You like to be the center of attention. Red portrays the adventurous side of you that's undeniable. Orange is texture and gutsy. Orange means you like to stand out in a crowd, never taking life for granted; you enjoy new challenges and have a tendency to come out on top. Yellow is always the optimist. You're athletic and outdoorsy. Yellow reflects a vibrant personality and great intuition.

Blue is fun-loving and free. Blue clothing attracts independent women who are comfortable with their inner selves and achievements. Those who favor white prefer safe colors for a perfect match. White can be a great accent for a deep, dark tan, adding sex appeal to the colorless color. If your heart's set on green, then you are a down-to-earth, natural beauty; while somewhat stubborn. You're still the girl next door, who likes to have fun and knows how to dress slimmer and look thinner.

Just remember, everyone's weight fluctuates, so mix and match your colors and accessories to your ever-changing body. While not everyone can be a size 6 or 8, the clothes you wear can make you look thinner, or have the opposite effect. It's your choice. You don't need to completely cover your body up if you have extra weight, and not every tip will work for you. You have some great features—accentuate them and accessorize. Find out what works best, flatter your figure, and stick with it.

A small weight gain will make your clothes feel tighter. Always have some "fat clothes" available for those occasions and don't feel bad. Every woman and man experiences this period. Dress slimmer and thinner with these modern fashion tips: Choose darker or solid colors such as black, navy blue, and gray. Dress monochromatic, in all in one color, top to bottom, no patterns. If you want to wear patterns, go for smaller ones that don't overlap. Avoid horizontal stripes. Look for thin vertical and diagonal lines for a fluid look. Select accessories to draw attention from trouble spots. Wear clothes that fit—not too baggy, but not too tight and clingy. Avoid bulky sweaters and sweatshirts. Always try on clothes before you buy them. Different designers have different size charts. Avoid pleats. Flat front pants and skirts are instant slimmers. Low-rise pants that fall just below your navel will highlight your torso. For longer-looking legs, skirts should fall right above the knee.

Forgo the frills. Extra ruffles and material only add bulk. If you have large breasts, it's best to buy a good support bra. Avoid shiny fabrics such as satin. High heels add shape to your legs. That's why you always see runway models in heels. Dark pantyhose will make large legs appear thinner. Stay away from patterned leggings. Wear undergarments such as control-top pantyhose and shapers. If you prefer wearing a sleeveless dress, cover your upper arms with the sheer elegance of a shawl. Choose an open-collar shirt and scoop necklines. Above all, avoid small handbags. Stick with a medium-size purse in proportion to your body.

A dress with a matching coat can hide bulges. Match your belt to your skirt or pants to make your legs appear longer. Don't tuck in your shirt. Let it fall just below your waist, but not too long, because it will make your torso appear short. You can still wear bright colors, just not on your problem areas. Frilly clothes are a no-no; they just add to your overall size. Avoid too-tight pants that cling to your hips and thighs. Instead, try trousers that will accentuate your legs with wide cuffs. For longer, thinner-looking legs, wear an asymmetrical tiered skirt. A straight waistline helps flatten the tummy.

It is also important for men to be knowledgeable about their clothing selection. Fashion tips and styles are not just for women. Men, wear your best—it will make you feel more confident in a business or social situation. How you present yourself correlates well with how you feel about yourself. If you don't appear to think much of yourself, don't expect others to. The women most men will want to meet in their professions know how a man should dress and are more attracted to one who meets those expectations. Most women know how to match colors. Brighter and edgier clothes and color combinations can work for men also, even at work; if your company is not too conservative. Primary bright colors can be mixed and matched and will stay in style for some time. Don't underestimate the versatility of black and white. Mixing black and white garments gives you a stunning variety of styles. You can put together more different color combinations with these two basic colors than with any others. You can also go monochrome, but take care that the shades match. To make your outfit a success, pair it with shirts and ties. If you go monochrome, pick a tie that is in a contrasting color. There is no such thing as a short-sleeve dress shirt, so don't wear it unless you have a suit jacket on top.

A white shirt with a dark suit is always safe for semi-formal evening wear; but always playing it safe is no fun either. Try a black suit with a colored shirt, such as dark red for change. At the office, white or blue dress shirts are business staples. Dark-tone, striped jackets will make a nice change. Opening your shirt collar and loosening your tie does not make you look cool or relaxed. Normally, you should wear a straight-collar shirt with a suit. A button-down collar dress shirt may be worn if it is of high quality, and button-downs also go nicely with a blazer or sport coat. Festive ties with teddy bears or Santa Claus faces are fine for festive occasions, but not for the office. Own at least two dress shirts of different colors with French cuffs. You can find cuff links that are color coordinated with your outfit at major department stores. If you are less than five feet ten inches, get a suit or blazer that has a short cut.

They are better proportioned for you. Never wear an armless muscle shirt outside the gym. Get rid of pants that taper at the bottom. They make you look top-heavy and overweight. Keep your pants pulled up. Be sure to buy a standard fifty-six-inch tie, unless you are over six feet tall or have a protruding belly.

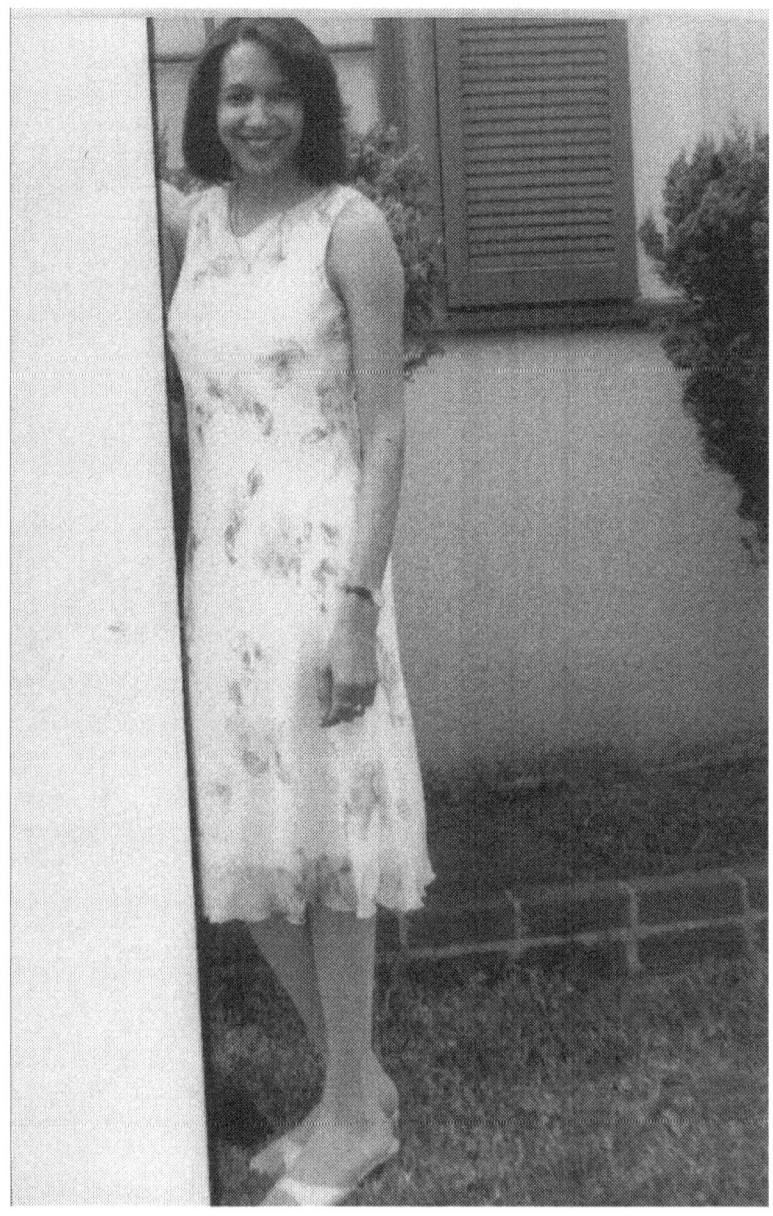

Easter Sunday – In my late thirties

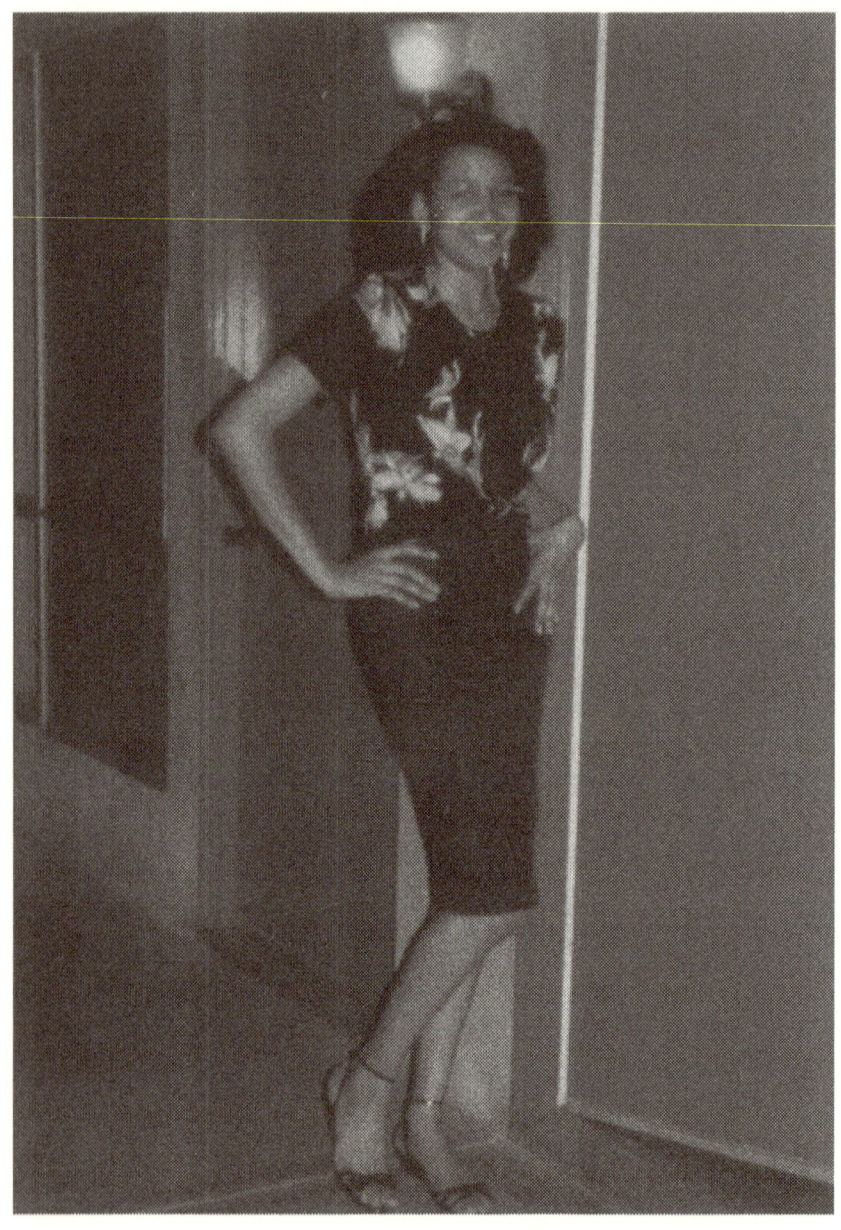

In my early twenties

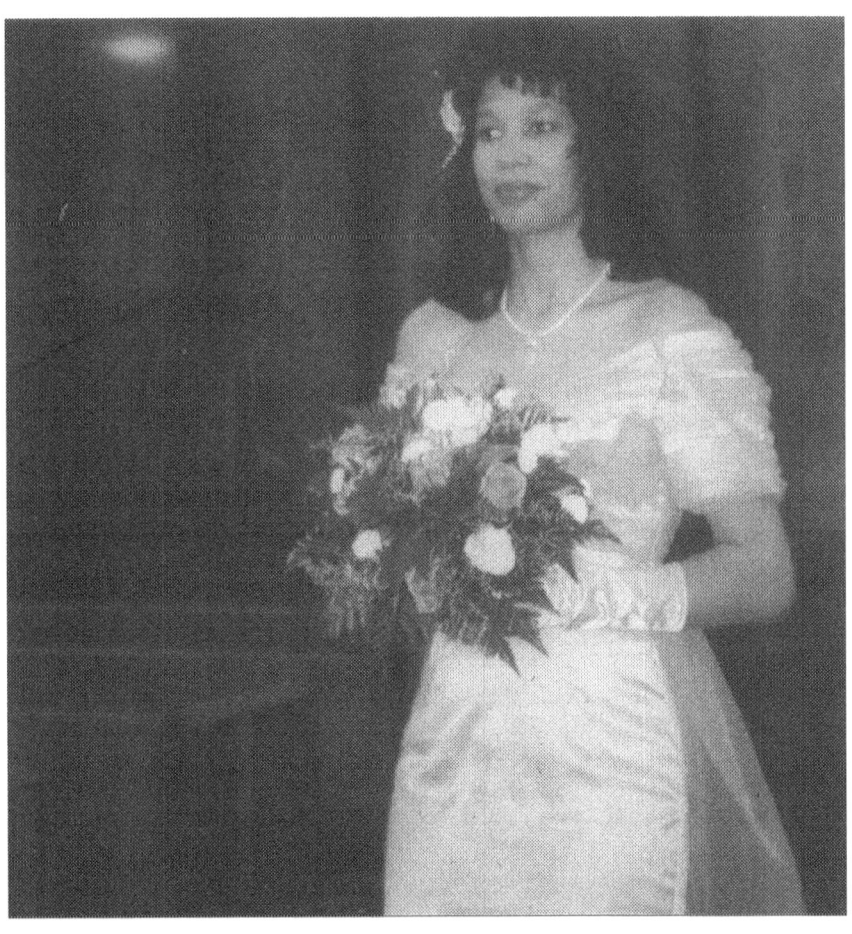

My sister's wedding – In my early thirties

CHAPTER 10

Learn to Love Your Body!
Maintain Confidence, a Positive Attitude, and a positive Self-image

     Everyone has a body image which affects the way they treat themselves and how they interact with loved ones. Often people judge their bodies based on this body image. This is often promoted by society and has unrealistic body images exhibited by models and promoted by Madison Avenue that overemphasize youth and attractiveness. Our responses to these societal pressures can be significant, especially with the increase in cosmetic surgery. People may be motivated to such actions for health reasons, yet how much more often are such risks taken out of a need for self-acceptance and self-love? Both of these qualities significantly impact a person's ability to establish and maintain healthy relationships with others. Family and romantic relationships are affected when we or the ones we love view our bodies in less than a healthy way. Twenty-four percent of women and 17 percent of men say they would give up more than three years of life to be thinner. That's according to a 1997 poll conducted by *Psychology Today* magazine. At the same time, studies show that half of American women overestimate the size of their bodies. So sociologists will study the Western world phenomenon of poor body image and attribute the problem to a variety of factors, including media, cultural influences, and peer pressure.

The advertising industry ties in the already complex issue of body image with materialism. A slender body is associated with wealth, health, and attractiveness. A heavier body is associated with loss, indulgence, and a lack of self-control. Psychological factors can also add to the effect of media, culture, and depictions of body image. Girls who experienced sexual abuse or who had an emotionally difficult puberty are more prone to body dissatisfaction as adults—so are women who feel they have little control over their lives. Women who have felt the most brutal blows from poor body image say that it is not caused by a single factor acting in isolation in regard to the dangers of body dissatisfaction. We realize that it is a combination of influences that lead to body dissatisfaction. But we can empower ourselves to solve the problem. We can use this power by breaking the chains of these influences, wherever we can. When someone has a poor body image, she will try to find validation from the outside to make herself feel better. The next guy, the next fashion fad, the next boyfriend. Anything but where they are now. Instead of living for tomorrow, it is time to start living for today and looking better. Remember, the goal of most advertising is to make you feel not okay, so that by using their product, you will become okay. I say: Start out with an "okay" feeling and then you'll buy only what you choose to have for yourself.

Most of us can think of a time when we thought that a new haircut, dress, or lipstick would turn everything around for us. But that mindset can lead to a lot of wasted time and money. Constant self-monitoring can also drain your energy and can even lead to depression and hostility. A University of Toronto study, published in the *International Journal of Eating Disorders*, found that women who were interviewed after seeing magazine ads that featured female models showed a significant decrease in self-esteem. Poor body image can lead to crash dieting and excessive exercise, which can in turn lead to poor nutrition, injuries, and depression. In its most dangerous form, a negative body image may fuel an eating disorder or *body dysmorphic disorder*, BDD. When you are continually distracted by thoughts of your physical appearance, the energy of your mind, body, and spirit is diverted from more serious endeavors. A more positive body image can help you in all of your roles. Improve your role as a mother by teaching your children how to love their bodies. Improve your physical health. Improve your role as a lover. One study showed that women who were comfortable with their bodies, regardless of size, achieved more sexual satisfaction than those who were more physically self-conscious.

If you feel that your body image has become a preoccupation, don't hesitate to talk to a counselor. Some people are too deeply entrenched in their body issues to consult a counselor on their own. Often, there are personal or family issues at play when a person has an eating disorder, so seeking professional help is highly recommended. Make small changes. A global changing culture and economic structure would no doubt help us all achieve a more positive body image. There will always be supermodels, paid endorsements, and the unstoppable quest for the best bandwagon. Instead, enforce changes on a smaller scale. We must stop allowing those negative forces into our lives. Don't buy *Cosmo*, buy *Redbook*. Look at really powerful, intelligent, successful women and men that you admire as often as possible, for example: Oprah, Hillary, Condoleezza, Colin Powell, your mom, your dad, your grandmother, grandfather, daughter, son, brother, sister, or friend. Seek out positive affirmations. When you catch yourself commiserating over tight blue jeans, don't let your mind get stuck in the negativity. When that negative voice does emerge, follow it with ten positive thoughts. Repetition is the key. Begin to re-record positive, pleasant messages over the negative messages in your own mind, which are so painful.

Once you navigate yourself out of the negativity rut, you'll feel better about yourself and you'll better understand your power to create and maintain a healthier mind, body, and spirit. Remember your spiritual connection. The first thing to remember is that God does not make mistakes. You are who you are for a reason. With this said; start to choose how to proceed with the next minute, hour, or day of your life. For those with a strong religious and spiritual sense, remember that your body image may not instantly improve with a simple reminder that God created your body for a specific purpose. He may not have made everyone to look like a gorgeous model, because each one of us is unique. He wants you to be healthy enough to do your life's work and to work at an optimal level; so accept his creation and nurture it. Gather with supportive friends. Surround yourself with them. Other women and men can make the biggest difference in your life by being mentors and leading by example. It is a good idea to find a group of women to be with regularly to discuss issues important to your life; but don't focus solely on body issues. Obsessing on things as a group is no better than obsessing as an individual.

Find a group of supportive women or men, either in your neighborhood or online. Then use and save non-critical articles to empower one another. Change the relationship with food. Food is fuel for active living. Strive not only for an ideal weight on the scale, but for a weight at which you feel strong and energetic. Teach yourself not to contribute to work that takes away from your health and energy levels. When we live without focusing on our bodies and begin to focus on our health, our bodies have an easier time finding our optimal weight. Researchers at the Stanford University School of Medicine have discovered that people who start a weight loss program when they feel happiest about their bodies are more than twice as likely to lose weight as people who aren't as satisfied.

I can't prove that we can control how much power food has over us, but one of the most important factors in my success has been to eat sensibly, in small portions, and not to deny any cravings. This sets my life up so that I don't ever feel needy for food. You can change your relationships with exercise and common-sense eating habits. Motivate yourself to exercise by reminding yourself about the burst of energy that inevitably follows a workout.

Change your relationship with food and your body will become a tool for increased strength and for making money. Suddenly, your body has the endurance and power to do whatever the mind wills. Our bodies are miracles, walking around in skin. You will never come across a finer work of art or machinery. The framework will allow you to ask yourself how you want to spend your energy. Imagine for a moment that you took all that time you spent thinking about appearance and focused on how much you love your ability to communicate well, or what a great mom, dad, sister, or brother you are. If you took the negative energy and used it for good, not only would you improve, but the world would improve as well. Your body is an ally in your life's work. Respect it as such. That is why it is important to have a healthy or positive body image. People have a healthy body image when they are comfortable with their bodies and have positive and self-confident feelings towards themselves. Research reveals that body image is also a major contributor to overall life happiness. This includes physical, psychological, and sexual aspects of life.

Body image forms early in life, in childhood, and adolescence. Physical activities impact later attitudes and behaviors related to the body. A recent study published in the *Journal of Social and Personal Relationships* found that body image of adolescents also affects the development of attitudes and behaviors associated with their romantic relationships. Their body image correlates with enhanced relations, connectedness, and attraction. What does it mean to have a negative body image? It means not liking your body, weight, or specific body parts. It may also include disliking your hair, skin color, or facial features. It's very common for women and men to have some degree of body image dissatisfaction. Generally speaking, sexuality, attractiveness, a weight concern, and physical condition all work together to produce a person's body image. Some of the things that may negatively affect body image are the influence of the media and popular culture, experiences of physical or sexual abuse, and a parent or loved one who is constantly preoccupied with his or her weight and dieting.

Being teased, bullied, or harassed based on size, skin color, or physical abilities can also make people have negative images about themselves. Physical changes in the body at different stages of life such as puberty and pregnancy, and even hair loss in middle-age, have been shown to be contributing factors. Participation in events in which extreme thinness is promoted, such as dance, gymnastics, and modeling, can put pressure on an individual towards crash dieting.

Ask yourself: How can I promote a healthy body image in myself? There is considerable evidence that body image can be influenced positively or negatively by external and internal factors. Ask a significant other to read and talk about this important health issue. Try not to use food as a reward or punishment.

Teach yourself to listen to your body and to trust its messages. It is okay to eat if you are hungry, even if it's not at meal time. Understand the nutritional and health benefits of various foods, instead of telling yourself that food is either good or bad. Compliment yourself and love your own strengths, accomplishments, and efforts, instead of focusing on weight size. People with unhealthy eating habits respond more to subliminal cues that emphasize fatness. With healthy eating habits, they can respond to subliminal cues that emphasize thinness.

Surround yourself with overt and subtle reinforcement for a positive body image. Friends who are uplifting and accepting of people will inspire you to take care of yourself and develop healthy eating habits and an exercise plan. If junk food must be kept in the house for others, putting it out of your sight and, hopefully, out of reach will help.

Play up the music at home. When you travel, sad songs can unconsciously motivate you to want to lift your mood with comfort foods. Make it a habit to drink water all day long, walk outside as much as possible, and enjoy learning to cook fun and healthy dishes at home—and play upbeat music while you do so. This technique of playing sexy music can be applied to any conscious effort you're making to enhance body image: exercising, cooking, drinking water, getting ready for a date, and reading magazines that feature realistic photos of men and women. The trick is, you want to start consciously and unconsciously associating your activities with as many positive stimuli as you can. Emphasize your favorite music or become attuned to other enticing sounds, such as trickling water or waves crashing on the shore, scents, and visual cues such as candles, certain colors, flowers, or mood lighting. In general, do all that you can to take care of your body. Always love and respect your body because if you don't, who will?

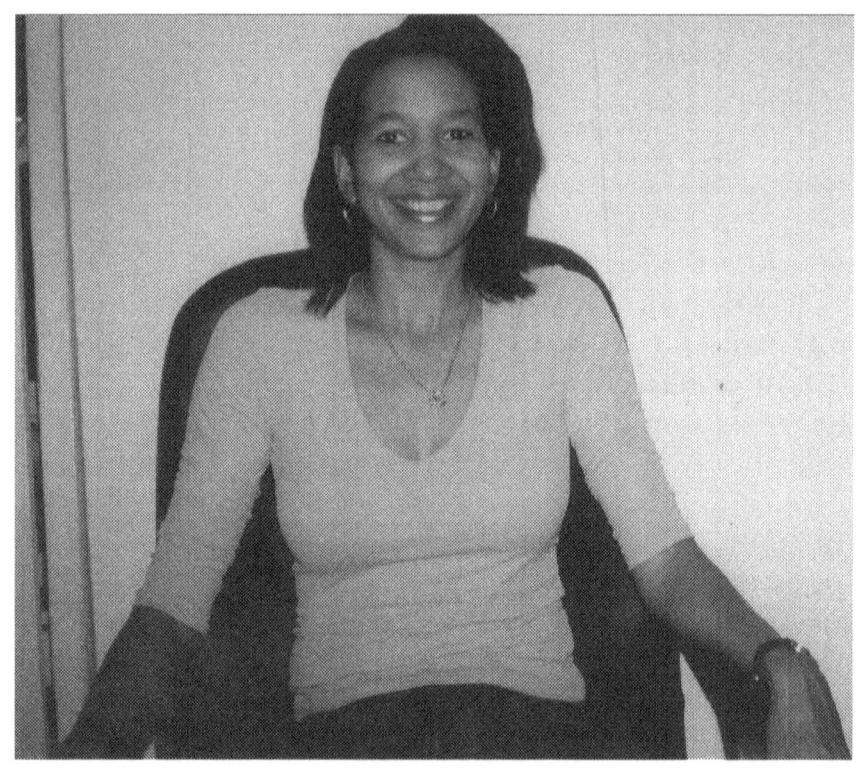

My son took this picture – In my middle thirties

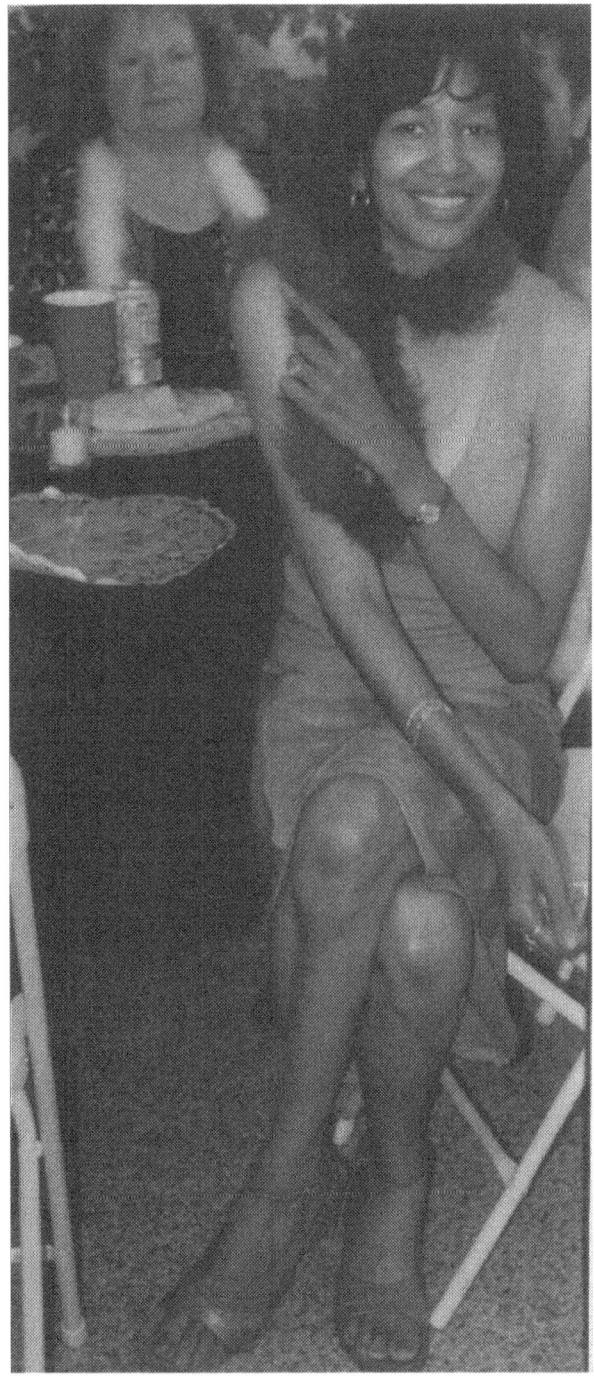

At a birthday celebration – In my early thirties

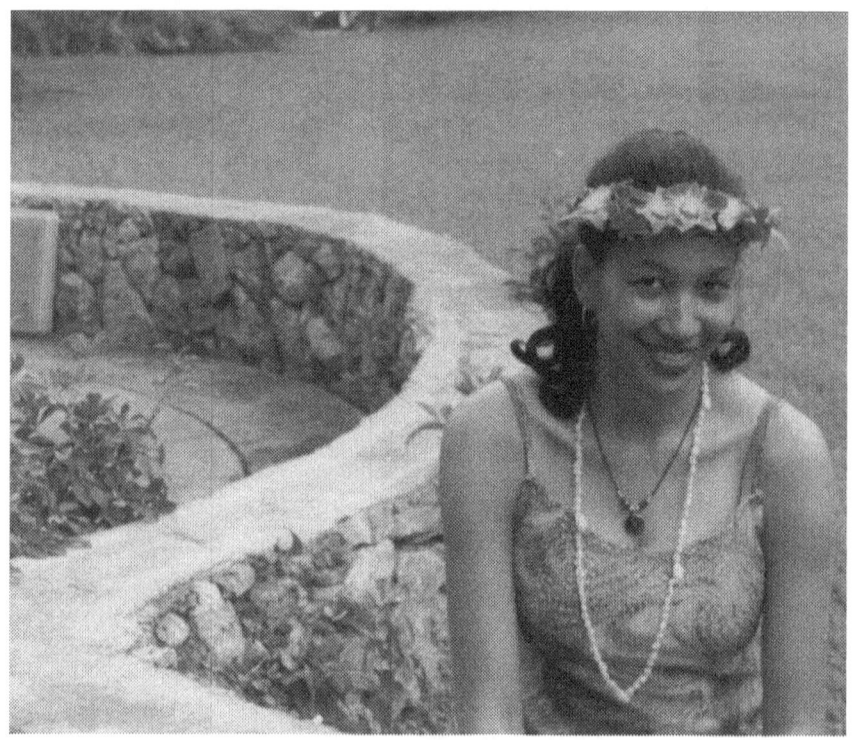

In Hawaii – In my late thirties

My wedding – In my late thirties

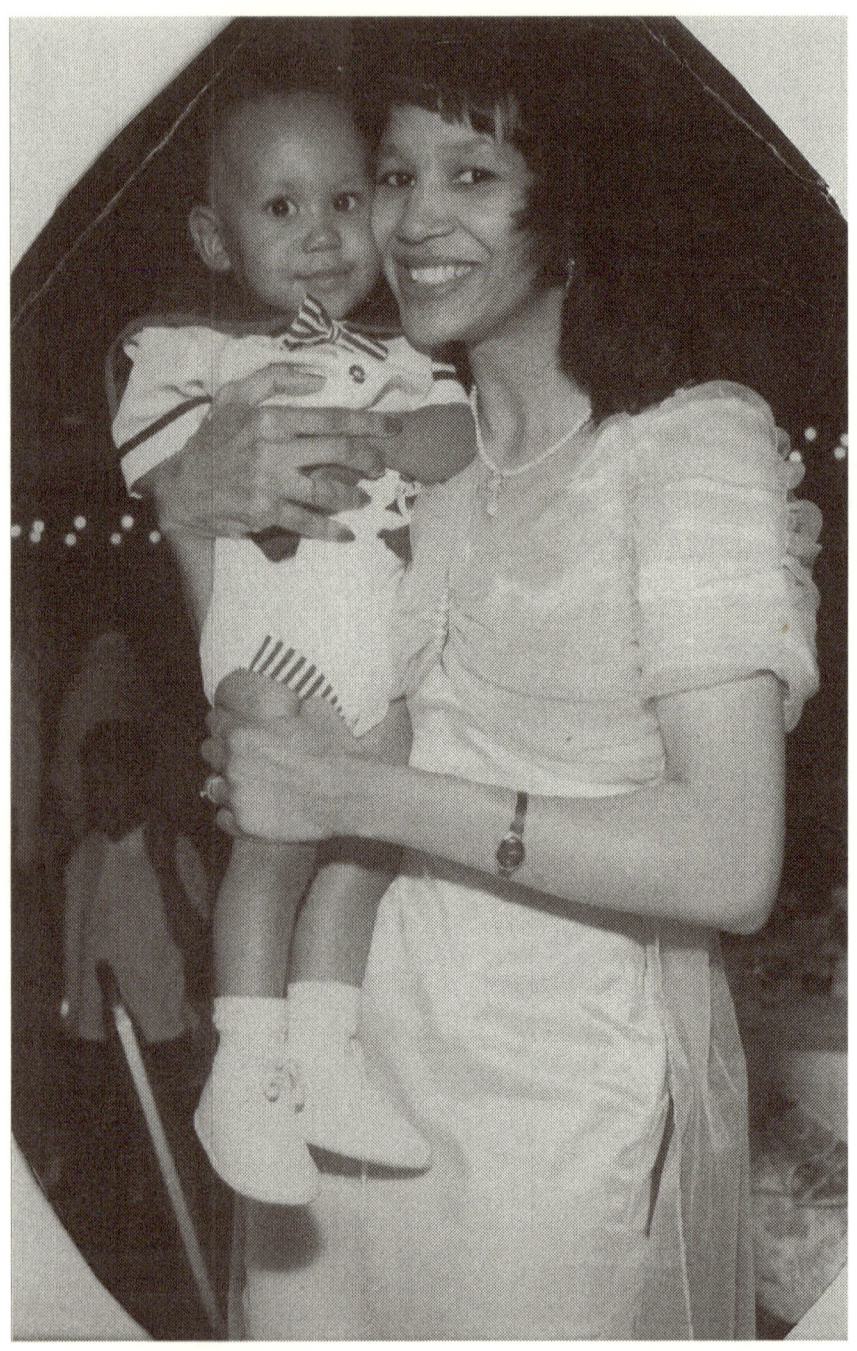

When my son was a year old – In my early thirties

www.ingramcontent.com/pod-product-compliance
Lightning Source LLC
Chambersburg PA
CBHW031325290526
45784CB00014B/1839